Bringing the Hospital Home

Recent and related titles in gerontology

Robert H. Binstock and Stephen G. Post, eds., *Too Old for Health Care?: Controversies in Medicine, Law, Economics, and Ethics*

Robert H. Binstock, Stephen G. Post, and Peter J. Whitehouse, eds., *Dementia and Aging: Ethics, Values, and Policy Choices*

Laurence B. McCullough and Nancy L. Wilson, eds., *Long-Term Care Decisions: Ethical and Conceptual Dimensions*

Harry R. Moody, *Ethics in an Aging Society*

Stephen B. Post, *The Moral Challenge of Alzheimer Disease*

Robert H. Binstock, consulting editor in gerontology

Bringing the Hospital Home

ETHICAL AND SOCIAL IMPLICATIONS
OF HIGH-TECH HOME CARE

EDITED BY

John D. Arras

H. WILLIAM PORTERFIELD, M.D., AND

LINDA OBENAUF PORTERFIELD

PROFESSOR OF BIOMEDICAL ETHICS AND

PROFESSOR, DEPARTMENT OF PHILOSOPHY

UNIVERSITY OF VIRGINIA

CHARLOTTESVILLE, VIRGINIA

The Johns Hopkins University Press
Baltimore and London

© 1995 The Johns Hopkins University Press
All rights reserved. Published 1995
Printed in the United States of America on acid-free paper
04 03 02 01 00 99 98 97 96 95   5 4 3 2 1

The Johns Hopkins University Press
2715 North Charles Street
Baltimore, Maryland 21218-4319
The Johns Hopkins Press Ltd., London

Library of Congress Cataloging-in-Publication Data will be found at the end
of this book.

A catalog record for this book is available from the British Library.

ISBN 0-8018-4990-X

Contents

List of Contributors. . . . . *vii*

Preface . . . . *xiii*

1. Introduction: Ethical and Social Implications of High-Tech
   Home Care   1
   JOHN D. ARRAS AND NANCY NEVELOFF DUBLER

   I. THE TECHNOLOGIES AND THEIR EFFECTS ON
      PATIENTS AND FAMILIES

2. The History of Respirators and Total Parenteral Nutrition
   in the Home and Their Use in Children Today 35
   ALEX OKUN

3. Chimeras and Odysseys: Toward Understanding the
   Technologically Dependent Child 53
   ARTHUR F. KOHRMAN

4. Oncology and High-Tech Home Care 65
   DAVID G. PFISTER

5. Issues in Long-Term and High-Tech Home Care for
   Persons with HIV Infection/AIDS. 79
   ANGELA MCCABE, JOSEPHINE PAREDES, AND DAVID G. PFISTER

6. Psychological, Social, and Ethical Issues in Home Care
   of Terminally Ill Patients: The Impact of Technology. . . 91
   SHERRY R. SCHACHTER AND JIMMIE C. HOLLAND

7. High-Tech Home Care for Elderly Persons: What,
   Why, and How Much? 107
   LIDIA POUSADA

8. High-Tech Home Care for Elderly Persons: Issues
   and Recommendations 129
   JEANIE KAYSER-JONES

II. PHILOSOPHICAL AND POLICY PERSPECTIVES ON
    HIGH-TECH HOME CARE

9. Moral Obligations or Moral Support for High-Tech
   Home Care? 149
   NEL NODDINGS

10. Transforming Homes and Hospitals 166
    WILLIAM RUDDICK

11. Problems and Protocols for Dying at Home in a
    High-Tech Environment 180
    MARSHALL B. KAPP

12. High-Tech Home Care in Context: Organization,
    Quality, and Ethical Ramifications 197
    ROSALIE A. KANE

13. The Economic Impact of High-Tech Home Care 220
    PETER S. ARNO, KAREN BONUCK, AND ROBERT PADGUG

14. Justice and Access to High-Tech Home Care 235
    NORMAN DANIELS

    Index 253

Contributors

Peter S. Arno, Ph.D., is Associate Professor of Health Economics in the Department of Epidemiology and Social Medicine, Montefiore Medical Center/Albert Einstein College of Medicine. Over the past decade, his work has focused on the economic and financial impacts of the AIDS and tuberculosis epidemics. Currently he is studying the regulation, innovation, and pricing practices of the pharmaceutical industry and the social and public health implications of regulating tobacco as a drug. Dr. Arno is co-author of *Against the Odds: The Story of AIDS Drug Development Politics & Profits.*

John D. Arras, Ph.D., is H. William Porterfield, M.D., and Linda Obenauf Porterfield Professor of Biomedical Ethics and Professor of Philosophy at the University of Virginia. (At the time of the preparation of this book he was Associate Professor of Bioethics at Montefiore Medical Center/Albert Einstein College of Medicine and Adjunct Associate Professor of Philosophy at Barnard College.) He is a Fellow of the Hastings Center and a former member of the New York State Task Force on Life and Law. Dr. Arras is the editor (with Bonnie Steinbock) of *Ethical Issues in Modern Medicine*, now in its fourth edition, and the author of numerous articles on bioethics. His primary areas of research include the forgoing of life-sustaining treatments, clinical issues in AIDS treatment and research, ethics and long-term care, and methodology in practical ethics.

Karen Bonuck, Ph.D., is Instructor in the Department of Epidemiology and Social Medicine at Montefiore Medical Center/Albert Einstein College of Medicine. Her research has primarily been on AIDS in families, health care, HIV illness affecting adults and children, the tuberculosis epidemics, and drug development and pricing.

Norman Daniels, Ph.D., is Goldthwaite Professor of Philosophy at Tufts University and Professor of Medical Ethics at Tufts Medical School. He has written widely on the philosophy of science, ethics, political and social philosophy, and medical ethics. His books include *Just Health Care* and *Am I My Parents' Keeper?: An Essay on Justice be-*

tween the Young and the Old, and he recently completed *Seeking Fair Treatment: From the AIDS Epidemic to National Health Care Reform.* A Fellow of the Hastings Center, Professor Daniels has lectured and consulted in the United States and abroad on issues of justice and health policy, including for the United Nations and for the President's Commission for the Study of Ethical Problems in Medicine.

Nancy Neveloff Dubler, LL.B., is Director of the Division of Bioethics, Department of Epidemiology and Social Medicine, Montefiore Medical Center, and Professor of Bioethics at the Albert Einstein College of Medicine. In 1978 she founded the Law and Ethics Consultation Service, which is available to all services and departments as a support for analysis in difficult cases. In 1980 she began the *Journal of Prision and Jail Health: Medicine, Law, Corrections, and Ethics.* She has lectured often about, and is the author of numerous articles and books on, the termination of care, home care and long-term care, geriatrics, prison and jail health care, and AIDS. Her most recent books are *Ethics On Call: Taking Charge of Life-and-Death Choices in Today's Health Care System* and *Mediating Bioethical Disputes.*

Jimmie C. Holland, M.D., is Chief of the Psychiatry Service at Memorial Sloan-Kettering Cancer Center and occupies the Wayne E. Chapman Chair in psychiatric oncology. She is senior editor of *Handbook of Psycho-Oncology* and co-editor of *Psycho-Oncology, the Journal of the Psychological, Social and Behavioral Dimensions of Cancer.* Dr. Holland has been active in the development of the subspecialty of psychooncology and in establishing national and international organizations to foster work in this field.

Rosalie A. Kane, D.S.W., is Professor of Public Health at the University of Minnesota, where she is also on the faculty of the Center for Biomedical Ethics and the School of Social Work, and she directs the Long-Term Care Resource Center. Her research focuses on health, personal care, and social services for elderly and other dependent groups, including the quality of care, assessment, case management, home care, nursing home care, and, more recently, the study of values and ethics. Dr. Kane is a past editor-in-chief of *The Gerontologist.* With Robert Kane, she coauthored five books: *Long-Term Care: Principles, Programs and Policies, A Will and a Way: What the United States Can Learn from Canada about Caring for the Elderly, Values and Long-Term Care, Assessing the Elderly: A Practical Guide to Measurement,* and *Long-Term Care in Six Countries: Implications for the United States.* With Arthur Caplan, she wrote *Everyday Ethics: Resolving Dilemmas in*

Nursing Home Life and *Ethical Conflict in the Management of Home Care: Case Manager's Dilemma.*

Marshall B. Kapp, J.D., M.P.H., is Professor in the School of Medicine at Wright State University, where he teaches courses on the legal and ethical aspects of health care. He is also director of the university's Office of Geriatric Medicine and Gerontology and holds an adjunct faculty appointment at the University of Dayton School of Law. Dr. Kapp is the author or coauthor of numerous articles, chapters, and reviews, and of seven books, including *Geriatrics and the Law: Patient Rights and Professional Responsibilities, Ethical and Legal Issues in Home Health Care,* and *Ethical Aspects of Health Care for the Elderly: An Annotated Bibliography.*

Jeanie Kayser-Jones, Ph.D., is Professor in the Department of Physiological Nursing, and in the Medical Anthropology Program, Department of Epidemiology and Biostatistics, School of Medicine at the University of California, San Francisco. She is also the Director of Graduate Studies in Gerontological Nursing. She has published widely in gerontology nursing, social science, medicine, and law journals and is the author of *Old, Alone, and Neglected: Care of the Aged in the United States and Scotland.* Dr. Kayser-Jones is recognized nationally and internationally for her reserarch in cross-cultural care of institutionalized elderly people, environment and aging, ethical issues in the care of elderly people, and the quality of care in nursing homes.

Arthur F. Kohrman, M.D., is President of La Rabida Children's Hospital and Research Center, the Pediatric Chronic Disease Center of the University of Chicago Department of Pediatrics, where he is also Professor and Associate Chair. Dr. Kohrman has been concerned for several years with the technological, psychological, economic, medical, and ethical issues surrounding the care of medically complex children at home and in the community. His broader interests are in the care of chronically ill and disabled children, in research relating to their medical care and the social barriers facing them and their families, and in the development of national policies to ensure that children with special health care needs are able to achieve the greatest possible success and security.

Angela M. McCabe, M.S.W., C.S.W., is Clinical Coordinator of HIV Social Work Services at Memorial Sloan-Kettering Cancer Center, where she is also Coordinator of the HIV Testing Program, a faculty member of the Psychosocial Oncology Institute, and a field instructor for master's-level social work students. She is Chairperson of the New York City Social Work AIDS Network and Chairperson of the Board of Directors of the Staten Island AIDS Task Force. She has lectured extensively throughout the country on the clinical perspectives of an HIV diagnosis, and examining the overall effect on individuals, couples, family, and society.

Nel Noddings, Ph.D., is Lee L. Jacks Professor of Child Education and Acting Dean of Education at Stanford University. She is a past president of the Philosophy of Education Society and president of the John Dewey Society. Her areas of special interest are feminist ethics, moral education, and mathematical problem solving. In addition to seven books—among them, *Caring: A Feminine Approach to Ethics and Moral Education, Women and Evil, The Challenge to Care in Schools,* and *Education for Intelligent Belief or Unbelief*—she is the author of more than one hundred articles and chapters on various topics ranging from the ethics of caring to mathematical problem solving.

Alex Okun, M.D., is Assistant Professor of Pediatrics at Albert Einstein College of Medicine and Medical Director of the Pediatric Outreach Program at the Bronx Municipal Hospital Center. This multidisciplinary program offers comprehensive primary care in the hospital and the home to children with complex chronic illness. It serves as a teaching site for medical students and postgraduate trainees in nursing and pediatrics. After medical school and pediatric training, and for two years before his current position, Dr. Okun was a general pediatrician in two Appalachian counties in southeastern Kentucky.

Robert A. Padgug, Ph.D., is Director of Health Policy and Government Affairs at Empire Blue Cross and Blue Shield, in New York City. He also has an appointment in the Department of Epidemiology and Social Medicine at Albert Einstein College of Medicine and has taught at the Robert F. Wagner Graduate School of Public Service, New York University, and at Rutgers University. He is the author of numerous articles on health care financing, health policy and reform, and HIV/AIDS.

Josephine Paredes, M.D., is Assistant Attending Physician of the Clinical Immunology Service at Memorial Sloan-Kettering Cancer Center and Instructor in Medicine at Cornell University Medical College. She is an oncologist primarily involved in the treatment of various stages of Kaposi sarcoma and in the use of biological agents to treat HIV infection and its manifestations.

David G. Pfister, M.D., is Assistant Attending Physician/Assistant Member at Memorial Sloan-Kettering Cancer Center and Assistant Professor of Medicine at Cornell University Medical College. He is a former Robert Wood Johnson Clinical Scholar and the recipient of an American Cancer Society Clinical Oncology Career Development Award. Dr. Pfister is a specialist in solid tumors, especially those involving the head and neck, and his research focuses on the development and outcome assessment of treatment strategies that preserve function and the quality of life.

Lidia Pousada, M.D., F.A.C.P., is Chief of the Division of Geriatrics and Gerontology at New Rochelle Hospital Medical Center and Associate Professor of Clinical Medicine at New York Medical College. She has published numerous articles on emergency geriatric care, the medical management of geriatric surgical patients, and the care of Hispanic elders. Her edited and coauthored books include *Geriatric Diagnostics: A Case Study Approach, Emergency Medicine for the House Officer, Emergency Nursing: A Practice Guide,* and *Case Studies in Emergency Medicine.* In addition to teaching and research, Dr. Pousada maintains an active primary-care geriatric practice, performing office evaluations and house calls.

William Ruddick, Ph.D., is Professor of Philosophy and Codirector of the Philosophy and Medicine Program at New York University. He has published on a range of issues involving patients, family members, and physicians, as well as on the teaching, consulting, and criticisms of philosophers in medical schools and centers. He coedited *Having Children: Philosophical and Legal Reflections on Parenthood* and edited *Philosophers in Medical Centers.*

Sherry R. Schachter, R.N., B.S.N., M.A., is Coordinator of the Psychiatry Home Care Program at Memorial Sloan-Kettering Cancer Center. She is currently working toward her Ph.D. in Thanatology. Ms. Schacter is a Certified Grief Counselor and has lectured and published numerous articles on psychosocial issues of dying patients, their families, and significant others.

Preface

What starker contrast might we imagine than that between hospital and home? We tend to think of hospitals as the exclusive bastions of acute, high-tech medicine: strange and forbidding places crammed with buzzing, beeping, flashing machinery. Presiding over this baffling scene are physicians and nurses, experts whose strenuous training has prepared them to be the sole dispensers of the medical mysteries. On the receiving end of this technological largesse is the patient, ripped from familiar surroundings of hearth and home, of kith and kin, truly a stranger in a strange land.

By contrast, we tend to think of the home as the place where we feel most "at home," most ourselves, a place where we are surrounded by familiar faces, furniture, sounds, smells, tastes, and the comforting rituals of everyday life (Mack, 1991). Home is a place far removed, both physically and emotionally, from the hospital, with its experts and their machines.

Or so we would like to think. In fact, however, during the past ten years the high-tech home care industry has rapidly and relentlessly erased, for increasing numbers of families, the boundary between hospital and home, between the intensive care unit and the living room. More and more patients now receive in the privacy of their homes highly sophisticated medical treatments—such as ventilator therapy and artificial nutrition channeled through infusion pumps—that twenty years ago would have been available only in special care units. Although most recipients of high-tech home care benefit from the periodic assistance of visiting nurses or home hospice workers, much of the time this high-tech care is dispensed not by physicians or other specially trained professionals but by patients themselves when capable, or by parents, spouses, adult children, and partners—that is, by ordinary people with no specialized medical training.

The growth of the high-tech home medical services industry has been explosive. In the space of a mere decade, high-tech home care has emerged from near total obscurity to become the fastest-growing sector of the entire health care economy, providing valuable benefits to hundreds of thousands of patients per year and earning billions of dollars for innovative and adventuresome companies. This phenomenal growth rate has been due to several factors. First and foremost were changes in federal reimbursement policies. As early as 1977, Medicare began to pay for home parenteral and enteral nutrition, but it wasn't until the advent of diagnosis-related groups (DRGs) and prospective payment for Medicare inpatient services in 1983 that the high-tech home care industry was launched on its current trajectory (OTA 1992). Hospitals suddenly had a serious financial incentive to discharge patients earlier than under the *ancien régime* of cost-based reimbursement. The earlier the discharge, however, the sicker patients tended to be. Many could not simply be discharged to home in the absence of continuing medical treatment for such conditions as serious respiratory or digestive disorders and certain chronic infections. For such patients and many others, the development of high-tech home care was the solution.

Medical manufacturers were soon developing increasingly sophisticated devices for the delivery of all manner of drugs, most requiring less space and less medical expertise to operate than standard versions. Given the manifest need, the technical means to meet it, and the promise of enormous profits, providers moved quickly to market devices, drugs, and ancillary services to hospitals, to insurance companies, and, in some cases, even directly to patients. Sorely neglected in this rush to profits, however, was any seeming awareness, let alone a systematic analysis, of the possible ethical impacts of these new developments on the patient, the family, and involved caregivers; the notion of "home" in our society; and the equitable extension of these new benefits. The symbiotic relationship binding the burgeoning high-tech home care industry and hospitals supported the escalating profits of the former and served the interests of the latter in early discharge, which in an era of prospective payment amounts to increased profits.

Another major reason for the boom in high-tech home care is that patients and families usually welcome this "technology transfer" from hospital to home. When things go well, high-tech home care can offer the best of both worlds: state-of-the-art medical technology deployed in the privacy of one's home by loving family and friends. For many parents, it is much better to have their ventilator-dependent child at home than in a faraway hospital; for AIDS patients and many others, to resume an otherwise normal life with the help of nightly TPN; for teens with cystic fibrosis, to attend school with the help of programable antibiotic infusion pumps; and for dying cancer patients, to receive adequate pain control amid familiar surroundings. As the father of a 13-year-old boy with cystic fibrosis put it, "Home health care has made the difference between day and night for [my son] Clay . . . If he has after-school activities, he just takes the pump along to school with him" (Freudenheim, 1988).

Yet, as we might have expected, a shadow looms over the upbeat rhetoric of medical progress. Notwithstanding all the undisputed benefits of high-tech home care for patients and families, we are gradually coming to see that these benefits are often freighted with problematic moral, social, and policy implications. Just as we have seen with the more familiar hospital-based technologies involving CPR, dialysis, and respirators, a significant gap is emerging between our home-based technical prowess and our ability to discern humane, just, and efficient uses of this technology. Increasingly, homes are becoming more like hospitals; esoteric technologies are imposing highly questionable burdens on patients and their families; relationships among physicians, nurses, and patients are being redefined; and medical interventions of unstudied, let alone unproven, efficacy are costing consumers and third-party payers billions in a "Wild West" environment of unregulated competition. Amidst all this frenetic expansion in the high-tech home care market, important questions bearing on access, equity, standards of quality, and the consequences of such care for patients and their families go largely unaddressed.

Clearly, it is time to take stock. In the spring of 1992, the Division of Bioethics and Health Policy of Montefiore Medical Center–Albert Einstein College of Medicine initiated a year-long research project entitled "The Technological Tether: Ethical and Social Implications of High-Tech Home Care." Our goals were to study the impact of high-tech home care on patients, families, and the provider-patient relationship and to recommend policies that might more adequately and justly regulate the dissemination of this technology. Toward this end, we assembled a working group of clinicians, scholars, and policy analysts for six days of intense discussions throughout the year. To put a human face on our deliberations, we invited several patients, family members, and involved friends to share with the group their experiences of high-tech home care. References to the cases of specific patients and their families are presented throughout the book, all pseudonymously, of course. To provide an adequate scholarly backdrop, we commissioned numerous papers both from outside experts and from within the ranks of the working group. Chapter 1 distills the main points that emerged from our collective deliberations.

Collaborative projects of this nature occasion numerous debts—

intellectual, logistical, and financial. First, I would like to thank Nancy Neveloff Dubler and Jeffrey Blustein, my colleagues and friends in the division of Bioethics and Health Policy at Montefiore–Einstein, for their helpful participation in various stages of this project. Nancy's energy, vast knowledge of long-term care, and commitment to social justice—and Jeff's philosophical collegiality and commitment to the highest standards of intellectual integrity—have both been a continuing source of inspiration to me. My other divisional friends, Douglas Shenson and Karen Porter came along too late to participate in the "Tech Tether Project," but they deserve thanks nonetheless for their sustaining intelligence and humanity.

This project was premised on the crucial contributions of the members of our working group. This company included not only the clinicians and scholars whose chapters grace these pages, but also several others who faithfully attended our meetings, made important presentations to the group, critiqued drafts of project documents, and informed our deliberations with their experience and insight. From this latter group I am pleased to acknowledge the contributions of Barry Bateman of Gouverneur Hospital; Ronald Bayer and Lawrence Brown of the Columbia University School of Public Health; Eileen Hanley, Bobbie Falls, and Patricia Dee-Kelly of Visiting Nurse Services of New York; Alan Fleischman, formerly of Montefiore–Einstein, and now at the New York Academy of Medicine; David Gould of the United Hospital Fund of New York; Jaber F. Gubrium, University of Florida; Alice Herb, SUNY Health Sciences Center, Brooklyn; Robert Klein of Montefiore Medical Center–Albert Einstein College of Medicine; Carol Levine of the Orphan Project, Fund for the City of New York; Mathy Mezey, School of Nursing, New York University; and Robert Stone of Blythedale Children's Hospital.

Heartfelt thanks are also due to the secretaries in the Division of Bioethics and Health Policy—Leslie Carrington, Wayne White, and Donele Harrison—for their expert assistance in preparing the grant application, helping to organize the project's meetings, and handling all the other innumerable details that make up this kind of ambitious, far-flung enterprise. Even during all-too-frequent periods of sustained panic and craziness in the office, our secretarial colleagues somehow managed to keep everything on an even and highly productive keel.

I would also like to thank the Oncology Center of the Johns Hopkins University School of Medicine for inviting me to deliver the David Barap Brin lecture in December 1992. Given the emerging centrality of high-tech home care for the field of oncology, I used that occasion to develop many of the ideas that took their final form in chapter 1 of this book. I am deeply grateful both to the faculty and medical students at Johns Hopkins and to Miriam and Louis Brin for their gracious hospitality and commitment to rigorous debate in medical ethics.

Heartfelt thanks are also due to Wendy Harris, Anne Schwartz, and Carol Zimmerman, our splendid editors at the Johns Hopkins University Press. Wendy adopted, supported, and helped to shape this project from the beginning, while Anne and Carol turned our rough manuscript into a highly polished text.

Finally and perhaps most importantly, it is a pleasure to acknowledge the farsighted and generous support of the Greenwall Foundation and the Commonwealth Fund in sponsoring and sustaining this project. William Stubing of Greenwall and Mo Katz of Commonwealth not only provided us with the requisite funding but also proved to be enormously helpful and enthusiastic collaborators at our working sessions. Although the project took much longer to complete than we had originally contemplated, I hope both of our sponsors will find this final product to have been worth the wait.

REFERENCES

Freudenheim, M. 1988. The Boom in Home Health Care. *New York Times,* 2 May, sec. D1, col. 4.

Mack, A., ed. 1991. Home: A place in the world. *Social Research* 58: 5–307.

U.S. Congress, Office of Technology Assessment (OTA). 1992. *Home Drug Infusion Therapy under Medicare,* p. 5. Washington, D.C.: U.S. Government Printing Office.

Bringing the Hospital Home

1. Introduction

ETHICAL AND SOCIAL IMPLICATIONS OF
HIGH-TECH HOME CARE

John D. Arras, Ph.D., and Nancy Neveloff Dubler, LL.B.

Perhaps the most striking thing about the phenomenon of high-tech home care is its complexity. During the past decade, a wide range of technical services has evolved to meet the needs of an equally wide spectrum of patient populations. The technologies encompass some relatively uncontroversial devices, designed to provide low-cost replacements for home health aides, such as personal emergency response systems and sensors that signal an alarm when the patient wanders beyond certain boundaries. Such innovations are usually modestly priced and offer significant benefits in terms of safety and peace of mind for both patients and families. Then there are relatively uncomplicated therapeutic measures, such as home oxygen dispensers, that provide important benefits—in this case, greater ease in breathing for a large population of elderly patients with compromised lungs—without imposing serious financial or management burdens on patients, caregivers, or society. Finally and most problematically, there are the paradigmatic "high-tech" therapeutic interventions that should be the main focus of ethical and social concern: sophisticated catheters and infusion pumps for the delivery of all manner of antibiotics, nutrition, and analgesics; home ventilator systems; and some extremely expensive but noninvasive hardware, such as the new Flexicare beds that relieve bed sores at a going rate of $20,000 per unit.

It is crucial to note at the beginning, however, that one cannot place a given technology anywhere on a spectrum of moral and social concern simply by referring to its status as "high tech." A great deal depends on the context of its deployment (i.e., on the "who," the

"where," the "why," and the "for how long," as well as the "what").
A wide variety of high-tech home care interventions is currently administered to a very broad spectrum of patients, including children,
elderly people, patients with cancer or AIDS, as well as a large number of otherwise completely functional, working adults. Whether a
given technology—for example, home ventilators—will tend to generate serious ethical and social problems depends on answers to a
large number of questions (e.g., Is the patient tethered to the machine
for a life of indefinite duration or only for a short time? Is the purpose
of the treatment merely palliative or is it meant primarily to restore
health or extend life? What is the quality of the life thus extended? Is
a family member or close friend present, able, and willing to shoulder
the burdens of care, and will he or she be available in the future as
the individual and collective situations change? If so, how great are
those burdens, given the level of care and the caregivers' other responsibilities? If no family member or friend is available, could care
be purchased to fill this management and supervisory void? Is the
home well equipped and clean, or, as is the case for many urban and
rural poor people, is it roach infested and lacking even "low-tech"
necessities such as telephone and refrigeration? And finally, what is
the cost of delivering this technology in this way, compared with
other ways in other settings?).

Despite the fact that the label "high tech" does not automatically
confer the status of "ethical/social problem" on any given procedure
or piece of medical equipment, it remains true that the phenomenal
growth of high-tech home care in the last decade poses at least one
novel problem and, like the AIDS epidemic, puts a distinctive spin
on older, more familiar problems. As we shall see in later discussions
of policy issues, still other problems, such as unabashed profiteering
by manufacturers and the failure of regulators and industry to assess
quality and efficacy, neither are new nor manifest a distinctive spin:
they are as familiar and American as apple pie.

If one were to ask what is really novel, from an ethical or social
point of view, about high-tech home care, we would respond that
it is the hypermedicalization of the home, the extension of medical
dominion to the heretofore private sphere of family and friends. In
the mid-1970s the social critic Ivan Illich warned of the dangers of
"social iatrogenesis," an inability to cope with our surroundings engendered in part by the medicalization of everyday life (Illich 1976).
Now, nearly twenty years later, Illich's misgivings would no doubt
be intensified were he to consider the phenomenon of high-tech
home care. Although the benefits of high-tech home care may often

outweigh the burdens to patients, families, and caring friends, the invasion of the home by high-tech medical procedures, mechanisms, and supporting personnel exerts a cost in terms of important values associated with the notion of home. How can someone be truly "at home," truly at ease, for example, when his or her living room has been transformed into a miniature intensive care unit?

Just as technology has a way of transforming human relationships, expectations, and the rhythms of everyday life in more institutional settings (Ellul 1964; Rhoden 1988; Winner 1977), we should expect it to have similar transformative effects in the home. Rooms occupied by the paraphernalia of high-tech medicine may cease to be what that they once were in the minds of their occupants; familiar and comforting family rituals, such as holiday meals, may lose their charm when centered around a mammoth Flexicare bed; and much of the privacy and intimacy of ordinary family life may be sacrificed to the institutional culture that trails in the wake of high-tech medicine. Skilled nurses must visit, instruct, and monitor the behavior of patient and family; precise schedules must be observed; and caregivers must contend on a daily, even hourly basis with complicated machinery and tubing, which might clog or break down at any moment. And after several decades of banishment to the hospital, death may eventually "come home," not in its formerly more benign manifestations, but with all the trappings of hospital-based medical and ethical bureaucracy. Family members may soon have to make room for risk managers in home deathbed scenes. (See chap. 11, this volume.)

Dying at home may be initially attractive in an abstract fashion to both patients and family members, but the reality is rarely benign. Agonal breathing, incontinence of urine and feces, and fear of impending death are facts about the dying process that have been largely hidden from Americans in an era when 80 percent of people die in hospitals and nursing homes. Moreover, the residue of the patient's death may distort future memories of the patient and of the room wherein he or she died. One friend of ours testifies that ten years after her husband's death from a brain tumor, she still avoids using the living room of their house, where his hospital bed was set up. Dying at home is thus a reversal of our cultural norm and may adversely affect the perception of spaces in the home long after the patient's death. Although family members might still have good reason to choose the option of dying at home for themselves and their loved ones, the possible long-range consequences should be a part of their decisional calculus.

The medicalization of the home is not, we would insist, the sort of ethical/social problem that fits nicely into the categories of "quandary ethics." Just as Daniel Callahan asked, in the context of the debate over health care priorities, "What kind of life?" (Callahan 1991), here we ask, "What kind of homes and families do we want our society to foster, and at what price?" Our problem is thus better described, not as an ethical "dilemma," but as a complex social phenomenon that improves life for many while threatening to erode for others the conditions that tend to foster important social goods and opportunities—such as a nurturing home life with its intimacy, privacy, and freedom from the bureaucratic and rationalized trappings of institutions, as well as full economic and social opportunities for women. While a Luddite response to high-tech home care is neither possible nor desirable at this point, the threat it poses to the conditions of a robust home life should inform decisions made by families and by social planners. All concerned should ask themselves under what conditions a household might cease to become a genuine home to anyone. Increased sensitivity to this sort of question might lead us as a society to explore other possible solutions, such as creating or reforming other institutions so as to make them more "homelike," rather than turning some homes into mere satellites of medical institutions.

The Impact of High-Tech Home Care on Patients and Families

The following case example illustrates the numerous benefits offered by high-tech home care.

> Mrs. Borrero, an elderly Ecuadorian lady with a dedicated and highly organized extended family living close by, had been fighting cancer for many years. Finally, it became clear to her physicians and to Mrs. Borrero that her cancer was rapidly advancing and that she would probably die within a year. Her medical requirements were fairly complicated, however, including a need for total parenteral nutrition (TPN). When the physicians suggested to family members that Mrs. Borrero might be cared for at home, they immediately welcomed the opportunity. Each member accepted a significant and well-defined role—for example, a daughter served as the primary "low-tech" caretaker, a granddaughter as the liaison with the medical professionals and dispenser of TPN—and together they cared for and treated Mrs. Borrero with great skill in a context of loving affection. The patient surely preferred this arrangement to the sterile confines of the hospital or skilled nursing facility, and her children and grandchildren derived enormous rewards and satisfaction as well. As her granddaughter, put it, "She was always there for us with love, support, and helpful advice. We're now giving back to her some of the love that she gave us."

Although the Borrero family may be exceptional in their degree of dedication, organization, and skill, their experience no doubt resonates with many family caregivers and recipients of high-tech home care. Many uses of high-tech home care are viewed by willing individuals and families as unalloyed benefits, as cherished opportunities to be with loved ones at home, rather than in a hospital, or to resume a normal life outside the home. In this section, we shall dwell on the darker side, investigating the more problematic implications of high-tech home care for both patients and caregivers. We examine a set of ethical and social problems that, while not being unique to high-tech home care, at least display a characteristic "spin" in this environment.

Problems of Meaning and Identity

While the following account of the "impacts" of high-tech home care lists its more problematic effects, not all of these are necessarily or uniformly burdensome. Some problematic impacts are simply ambiguous, posing problems of meaning and identity for individuals, families, and even (as we have just seen) homes.

Some individuals receiving high-tech care complain about being "tethered" to a machine for a significant portion of each day. They wonder, "What have I become? What happened to that other self that was unencumbered by tubes and machines?" For some patients, resort to high-tech home care may result in a distorted body image that erodes self-esteem. ("I can't be seen in public with this machine always strapped to my shoulder.") For others, however, life with a high-tech device may be viewed as a challenge or even as an adventure. Some early patients on portable home ventilators described themselves as "respinauts" (Goldberg 1983)!

Problems of identity may be especially acute and far-reaching for children and adolescents, particularly for those tethered to a respirator for most, if not all, of their daily lives. What are we to make of the fact that a child beginning life with damaged lungs must have a constant mechanical companion? What does the child make of this dependence and interpenetration of identity? What are the boundaries, both physical and psychic, between child and machine (see chap. 3, this volume).

Families and close friends are constantly confronted with perplexing, challenging, and changing problems of identity in the course of caring for loved ones on high-tech home care. As sociologist Jaber Gubrium felicitously put it, home care is "biographical work." It is work that often challenges us to redefine our relationships with others and our images of ourselves; it is work fraught with the construction of meaning, not just with predefined "burdens" or "benefits." Thus, as an elderly or AIDS-afflicted loved one slowly slips into moderate, then severe dementia, the caregivers may wonder, "What has become of my spouse (friend, lover)? Is this still the same person I lived with and cared about, or is this a different person entirely, a stranger who no longer acknowledges me and whom I no longer recognize?"

Individual family members caring for loved ones regularly confront similar questions bearing on their own identity and social roles. Parents caring for technology-dependent children naturally wish to maintain and foster an exclusively loving, nurturing, and comforting relationship with their child. Their natural role is to protect, to safeguard from harm, to reassure. But these same parents, in their role as dispensers and maintainers of high-tech medical treatments, must sometimes inflict serious pain and suffering on their own children. In this second role, they must act more like doctors than parents, more like technicians than nurturing mothers and fathers. At such moments, they must often wonder "What am I doing? What have I become?" Indeed, many may well wonder whether their ventilator-dependent children might be better off elsewhere, perhaps in a comfortable residential setting, so the child might focus his or her inevitable rage against others and the family members might be better able to retain their identities as caring nurturers.

The experience of high-tech home care may prompt questions about identity and purpose for entire families. For Mrs. Borrero's family, providing TPN at home proved to be an immensely rewarding challenge. They may have overcome any residual doubts about their individual or collective commitments and risen to the occasion with a resounding rhetorical question, "What kind of family are we, anyway?" Other, less resourceful and less fortunate families must often ask themselves in the midst of exhaustion, fear, and despair, "What is happening to us? Are we still a family in any sense of the word, or have we all been reduced to the status of harried care providers, ourselves tethered to the machines and their implacable demands?"

Burdens to Caregivers

Caring for a family member or close friend on high-tech home care can be extremely demanding. Even without the addition of any complex machinery or procedures, the business of providing home care can be difficult and at times overwhelming for nonprofessional providers (Kane and Reinardy 1990). These unpaid family members or close friends must often provide such services as personal care (bathing, dressing, toileting, cooking and feeding, lifting, etc.); household chores such as laundry, house cleaning, and yardwork; transportation and help with errands outside the home; general supervision; and rudimentary medical care (injections, dressing care, medications, etc.). Add to all this the considerable complexity and difficulty of administering high-tech medical care, and the burden can become formidable indeed.

First, caregivers must learn a great deal about the relevant technology (for example, how to unclog catheters, suction secretions, prepare TPN solutions, and troubleshoot faltering equipment). These are all complicated, difficult skills that not so long ago were the exclusive province of trained medical personnel. It can be extremely intimidating for family members without a medical background to have to master the intricacies of these techniques in a relatively short time before hospital discharge, and then to be responsible when the patient is sent home. Many caregivers, for example, can be easily confused and threatened by complex gadgetry, while the parents of chronically sick and home-bound children often live with the constant threat of mishap and panic. "What if something goes wrong? What if the machine stops working? What will I do?"

Thus, the transition from hospital to home can be experienced by both patients and family members as a shift from what might be called technological overload to technological isolation at home. In the hospital, patients and families are surrounded by an intensely high-tech environment, including highly skilled support staff always just a call bell away. Patients not only receive treatment but also benefit from a highly routinized schedule of diagnostic tests that closely, accurately, and constantly monitor their status. At home, by contrast, some patients and their families can feel cut off from or even abandoned by this system of intensive medical supports. Physicians don't usually make home visits and, since they don't get reimbursed for long phone conversations, the close ties uniting them to families are often severed at discharge. Families can experience this lack of connection as a profoundly alienating and isolating experience. Thrown back on their own resources and instincts, families must often rely on impression and guesswork rather than data. The ensuing magnification of uncertainty can be a source of great worry and anxiety.

Apart from the difficulty of learning how to provide high-tech home care, there is the sheer magnitude of the amount of caring required. While this naturally varies from patient to patient and from one high-tech device to another, in many cases the burden can be significant and, in some cases, overwhelming. For some categories of patient (e.g., elderly persons with dementia, patients with cancer or AIDS) the primary source of the difficulty of providing care may lie not so much in the technological hardware, although that too can be formidable, as in the pathos of the disease's inevitable trajectory. It is just plain hard work to provide round-the-clock care for dying patients, especially for those who have lost control of their bodily functions. In such cases, the high-tech dimension might "merely" exacerbate an already difficult and stressful situation.

In other cases, however, the technology is itself largely responsible for the social stress; without it, the patient would never have lived long enough to come home. We think here, for example, of the parents caring for ventilator-dependent children. As opposed to patients with cancer or AIDS, whose impending death will eventually bring closure for stressed caregivers, ventilator-dependent children can signify a lifetime of demanding responsibility for parents. As Arthur Kohrman observed, for such parents the sense of "endlessness" can be overwhelming (Corbin and Strauss 1988; Kohrman 1991).

Any account of the burdens borne by caregivers must emphasize the fact that they do not fall evenly or haphazardly on family members. With the prominent exceptions of husbands who care for their cancer-stricken wives and an increasing number of gay men attending to their partners suffering from AIDS (Monette 1988; van den Boom 1991), this is for the most part work that women do: wives of chronically ill husbands, adult daughters of elderly parents, and mothers of technologically dependent children. The prevailing attitude seems to be, "Women are good at this sort of thing; and besides, if they are already at home, surely they can always make room for one additional responsibility." This attitude is graphically and unselfconsciously displayed in a widely published advertisement for the Aetna insurance company. Beneath a small child's colorful drawing of the whole family—including Mom, Dad, daughter Lisa, and Lisa's doll—we read the following copy: "When Lisa was born her kidneys didn't work. So we helped Lisa's mother learn to care for her . . . It saved $200,000 in hospital costs . . . And let Lisa grow up at home." One wonders why Aetna's "individual case managers" didn't also teach Lisa's dad to care for her, and whether Lisa's mom had to give up her job or career to save the insurance company so much money.

Our rosy picture of "home" is thus often parasitic on widespread but socially unjust roles for women caretakers. The traditional image of the "home as castle" reflects a male point of view; its appeal derives in large measure from the unstated premise that *someone else* will be doing the cooking, cleaning, and caregiving. In most cases, that someone will be a woman.

Although many women come to regard these burdens, which can sometimes be all-consuming, as opportunities for reciprocity or gratitude (recall Mrs. Borrero's family), others may come to see their lives reduced, not so much by choice as by circumstance, solely to the status of nurse and maid. For in addition to the constant stresses and strains of providing care on an hourly basis, there are serious opportunity costs: women charged with the care of ventilator-dependent children, for example, must usually forsake any possibility of work or professional satisfaction outside the home. They may be so immersed in giving care and tending machines that they effectively cease to have projects and lives of their own.

Failures of the Delivery "System"

Caring for ailing family members, partners, or close friends at home will always entail a certain amount of extra stress and burden, and caring for those with high-tech needs will usually increase the level of anxiety and difficulty. These inevitable burdens are, however, considerably exacerbated by deficiencies in our current system, really a nonsystem, of delivering high-tech home care.

The first problem, involving deficiencies of communication, arises at the stage of discharge planning in the hospital. Patients and their future caregivers often do not receive adequate instruction on how to perform high-tech procedures and are often ill-prepared for the magnitude of the task at hand (See chap. 8, this volume).

Second, patients and caregivers often confront a fragmented and bewildering maze of vendors, insurance companies, and nursing agencies. The experience of Mr. Chao is fairly typical in this regard.

Mr. Chao's wife, aged 59, was discharged from the hospital with phlebitis related to metastatic cancer that proved refractory to the customary anticoagulant approaches and required a continuous infusion of heparin. A chest port provided an access point for the drugs, which were delivered through a high-tech infusion pump. While this device made travel possible, it posed various problems. According to Mr. Chao, his wife had to be treated at home for two episodes of infection due to the device. In addition, he noted that few nursing agencies had the requisite skills for this kind of technologically sophisticated machinery. One agency said that they would manage her care but later reneged. While Mrs. Chao was receiving intravenous heparin therapy, the vendor sent six different nurses in the course of a single week, one of whom didn't know how to operate the pump. In addition, the vendor's nurses were not authorized to draw blood for needed tests, a service Mr. Chao had to pay for separately.

Mr. Chao found himself constantly on the phone with numerous vendors and agencies, who provided him with precious little information on costs, coverage, and payment mechanisms. (The infusion pump rental actually cost $150 per day. Over and above his bills for nursing services, which were considerable, Mr. Chao's total "high-tech" charges amounted to $18,000 at the end of four and a half months. Fortunately, through the intercession of his children, this bill was eventually reduced by two-thirds.)

This caregiver thus found himself in the unenviable position of actually having to *shop* for services without any reliable knowledge bearing on either quality or cost. In other cases, ambitious vendors have actually resorted to directly contacting elderly patients and their families, trying to "sell" them and their doctors on the need for high-tech devices and services (Pear 1991). Although some people believe that the free market should drive all transactions in health care, Mr. Chao's experience and that of many others must have been more akin to shopping blindfolded in a foreign bazaar than to the theorists' ideal market.

It is certainly true that technical supports, such as paid caregivers, are often available to families and that families sometimes have help in shouldering the burdens of high-tech home care. The troubling point, however, is that these supports are rarely organized into an efficient, coherent, and comprehensive package that provides a sense of security. (One project participant commented in this connection that users of WordPerfect, a popular word-processing program, often get more psychosocial support than the recipients of high-tech home care.) Patients and families often spend an inordinate amount of time, often putting their day "on hold," just waiting for nurses, aides, or vendors to return calls or show up. In addition, they have to *coordinate* the care provided by all of these parties, a time-consuming task that requires great skill and patience.

This void in patient management is rarely adequately filled either by home care agencies or by visiting personnel. Indeed, those who provide technical support are often employed by vendors of high-tech equipment in pursuit of a very narrow agenda—the accumulation of profits—that has little to do with the provision of truly comprehensive care. In contrast to hospice care, which prides itself on serving and supporting families with targeted case-management services that identify and coordinate all the complex elements of a comprehensive home care plan, high-tech home care is animated by no such holistic vision. All too often the case manager in high-tech arrangements tends to be the primary family caregiver.

Another major inadequacy of the current nonsystem lies in its failure to provide intermediate institutions between the hospital and home. Currently, many patients and their caregivers can choose between only hospital and home; between a highly regimented, alienating institution that can easily meet all their high-tech needs and the fragile comforts of home, where the demands of high-tech care can exhaust and overwhelm everyone concerned. And, as previously noted, given the pressure of diagnosis-related groups (DRGs) to discharge patients from the hospital, a "choice" between hospital and home may not even exist for many families.

Even where there is a real possibility of a technology-dependent patient remaining in a hospital or long-term care facility, the choice between institution and home may be more illusory than real. Consider the "choice" currently imposed on the parents of ventilator-dependent children. When asked by trusted pediatricians whether they would "like" to have their child go home, parents have no choice but to accept the burdens of home care. To say "no" would most likely be interpreted by others as evidence of a lack of caring and commitment; those who refuse might be labeled "bad" parents. Thus, the parents cannot effectively refuse to bring their children home, yet the cost to them is often crippling, in both personal and economic terms. Clearly, in many cases such parents are in a no-win situation.

In sum, then, we can say that the burdens to caregivers imposed by high-tech home care will vary with the level of technological intensity, the duration of care, and the presence or absence of good communication, case management, and intermediate institutions. Thus, a brief, well-managed regimen of palliative home care for a dying cancer patient might offer significant benefits to patient and family and present a manageable burden, while the chronic, long-term care of a ventilator-dependent child with limited possibilities for growth and development could easily fall on the other end of the spectrum, especially in the absence of meaningful social supports.

It is true that many of the problems enumerated above are not, strictly speaking, especially novel. Some of them merely appear to be high-tech versions of equally serious problems encountered in low-tech settings. For example, caring for a progressively declining patient with Alzheimer disease at home can give rise to the same feelings of alienation and endlessness, to the same challenges to personal and family identity, and to similar burdens to the family as the chronic care of a ventilator-dependent child. In many instances, then, it would not be wrong to argue that the major ethical issue isn't necessarily the high-tech component, but rather the chronicity, the intensity, and the emotional, economic, and social costs to the family and caregivers.

Despite these commonalities that cut across the high- versus low-tech dichotomy, we would insist that high-tech home care tends to generate these problems with ever greater frequency and intensity for more and more families. Although high-tech interventions do not necessarily impose excessive burdens on caregivers and patients, their very nature as high tech introduces elements that tend to impose burdens. Patients with high-tech needs tend to be sicker—fifteen years ago, many would have died much sooner from their underlying conditions; the rest would have remained confined in hospitals or nursing homes—and naturally will need more attention than many other categories of chronically ill, home-bound patients.

In addition, the availability of high-tech home care places ordinary people with no medical background, many of them elderly, in the stressful position of having to master fairly complicated technical regimens. In the event of malfunction, caregivers must be able to respond immediately, just as they do in the intensive care unit, to prevent serious damage or even death. What if the respirator fails, the catheter clogs, or the arterial line breaks or becomes infected? In the home, there is no nursing station down the hall; even when things are going well, many caregivers must constantly worry that they *might* go wrong at any time. Then there is the added stress of specialized medical personnel, volunteers, and others coming into the home to perform especially difficult tasks and to monitor the patient's care, often severely eroding familial privacy and intimacy in the process. In combination, all these problematic factors make high-tech home care a social phenomenon worthy of ethical reflection in its own right.

Health Care Providers, Patients, and Family Caregivers

The rise of high-tech home care poses serious and interesting challenges to our understanding of the complex network of relationships binding nurses, doctors, technicians, patients, and families. According to the relationship model developed in the context of acute care, hospital-based medicine, the physician gives the "orders" to nurses and patients. Insofar as we speak of a health care "team," the physician is indisputably the captain of that team. The role of the family in this context has been largely, in theory at least, to support and encourage the patient, engaging in decision making only when the patient lacks capacity because of age (e.g., minors, elderly people) or illness. Physicians and hospital administrators generally treat conflicting interests (for example, among family and patient) as "conflicts of interest" that tend to disqualify families from assuming decision-making roles (Arras 1995).

The home care setting presents an entirely different constellation of social relationships, challenging us to reconceptualize the dominant model of the patient-doctor relationship. Since the mid-1940s, physicians have been gradually but steadily fading from the home care picture. Because of concerns about poor reimbursement, time inefficiency, legal liability, and their ability to deliver high-quality care in the absence of reliable diagnostic, technical, and nursing supports, physicians have retreated to their offices and hospitals as the preferred sites of health care delivery (AMA 1991; Siwek 1989).

The resulting power vacuum has been filled by a wide variety of home care "players," including nurses (nurse practitioners, licensed practical nurses, registered nurses), home care agencies, technicians, home attendants, social workers, and case managers. For their part, patient-clients and their caregiving family members have a different status at home from that in the hospital. No longer passive "strangers in a strange land," the patient and family have legitimate and powerful interests deriving not only from the fact that they are now on their own turf but also from their active participation in the delivery of care.

In stark contrast, then, to the model of physician dominance conveyed by the "team captain" metaphor, authority and responsibility are widely dispersed and shared in the home setting. Recognizing this diffusion of power and authority as a *fait accompli*, the American Medical Association recently called on physicians to play more of "an active and major role on the home health care team"—not the *dominant* role usually coveted by the AMA— and to help forge a more collaborative model of interaction among health care professionals (1991, p. 771). Power and authority have been so widely fragmented, in fact, that often no one is in charge and responsible for the overall direction and daily management of some home patient-clients' care.

Physicians' worries about loss of control over the quality of care are particularly pertinent in the high-tech home care setting. It's one thing to retreat to the sidelines when the care provided by others at home is either decidedly low tech (e.g., changing bandages) or "no tech" (i.e., largely custodial services such as cooking, cleaning, shopping, etc.); it is quite another thing, however, when the responsibility for the use and maintenance of ventilators and infusion pumps falls into the hands of largely unskilled and unsupervised family caregivers. The emergence of high-tech home care as a widely available option thus poses profoundly difficult questions for physicians who are cognizant of the benefits of home care yet reluctant to cede the control of highly sophisticated technologies (Lantos and Kohrman 1992).

What, for example, is in the "best interests" of a child on the cusp of discharge to home care on a ventilator? The interpretive meaning of this important concept obviously depends on one's point of view. For many patients and family members, the ability to return home and stay there assumes enormous significance, so much so that they are prepared to view just about any home care plan, even those posing significant medical risks, as being in the child's overall best interest. Given the important role of home space in providing a sense of well-being and conditions for nurturing psychological growth, this is not an obviously irrational or neglectful point of view. But for many physicians who are more "at home" in the hospital, whose standards of appropriate care have been forged in the exacting environment of the intensive care unit, the child's best interests might be better served by highly skilled and dependable medical personnel working in well-equipped institutional settings.

Clearly, both of these perspectives on the child's best interests have merit, and families and physicians will have to work together to forge a new, more encompassing vision of high-tech home care collaboration. Surely families are correct in advancing a more holistic definition of best interests, one that incorporates a concern not merely for acceptable "laboratory values" but also for the child's emotional growth and socialization. But caregiving family members must nevertheless remain alert to the distinction between a reasonable desire to keep a child at home and a well-motivated but neglectful failure to report potentially life-threatening conditions to physicians. Because of their distance from the site of care, physicians involved with high-tech home care are especially dependent on families for openness and truthfulness; while family members, because of their unfamiliarity with the workings and implications of high-tech interventions, are especially dependent on physicians for full disclosure of the range of benefits and burdens of high-tech care at home.

As they engage in these discussions with family members, the hospital staff—especially physicians, nurses, and social workers—should be acutely sensitive to the dangers of double agency. As hospitals move to minimize their losses from extended lengths of stay and seek to penalize "offending" physicians, and as social workers are increasingly rated on the success of their discharge plans, there are escalating incentives for professionals in these positions to subtly shade the discussion to encourage speedy discharge. Just as fee-for-service medicine has always tempted physicians to provide unnecessary care for financial gain, the new cost-containment structures generate precisely the opposite motive, tempting discharge planners to benefit the hospital at the possible expense of unsuspecting families. Given their fiduciary relationship with patients and their families, health care professionals have an obligation to resist this temptation.

Time and money pose additional obstacles to physicians' full participation in high-tech home care. The care of chronically ill and technologically dependent patients can be extraordinarily time-consuming, especially when home visits are a central part of the discharge plan. Because of the exigencies of their busy practices, many physicians do not feel that they can or should commit large blocks of time for this purpose. In addition, many insurance plans currently deny physicians reimbursement for time spent on the phone with families or managing a home care plan (Larkin 1992).

This disenfranchisement of physicians from the delivery and management of home care is especially problematic when high-tech care is involved. While managing the chronic care of a patient whose condition is stable may require only the intermittent attention of a primary care physician or subspecialist, patients on high-tech home care have often been discharged from the hospital quicker, sicker, and in less stable conditions. Diseases like AIDS are by definition dynamic and need the close supervision of a highly trained physician knowledgeable about the latest reports of successful protocols. To the extent that home care patients receive highly complex and medicalized treatments for potentially volatile conditions, physicians should be involved in their care in a serious and ongoing fashion, even if not as captains of the team. Ways will have to be found, then, to minimize such obstacles to physicians' participation in high-tech home care.

Those who have delivered high-tech care in the home attest that this kind of practice can bestow significant rewards and satisfactions on health care professionals. In the home one sees more than a minuscule slice of the patient's dislocated life in a doctor's office; one sees the patient surrounded by "lived space," by family and friends, and by photographs of the patient's earlier life and relationships. As one nurse put it, "All hospitals are alike, but each home is different." Through home visits, one can discern not only the positive factors that must be galvanized into a coherent plan of care but also on occasion why some homes are not hospitable to particular patients. If physicians, nurse practitioners, and others are to establish successful collaborations with patients and their caregivers, they must understand these various relationships and the dynamics they foster.

The rise of high-tech home care poses different challenges for nurses. While physicians tend to experience the shift from hospital to home care as an alienating loss of control, many nurses embrace high-tech home care as a liberation from the constraining rules and roles of the hospital. Nurses often complain that in the hospital they bear many responsibilities but are granted little, if any, authority or discretion. Physicians give orders, and nurses follow orders to the letter. In the home care setting, by contrast, nurses assume a heavy load of responsibility, but they also tend to be granted more authority, even if only by virtue of their distance from the hospital and greater flexibility in carrying out the plan of care. To be sure, delivering high-tech care in the home can involve treacherous family dynamics, complicated medical regimens, sophisticated machinery, crushing caseloads, and "jerry-rigged" extension cords. Juggling all these factors is no doubt difficult and emotionally taxing work, but for many nurses who deliver high-tech home care, such problems are also invitations to a much more independent, creative, and satisfying model of nursing care.

The Decision for High-Tech Home Care: Medical and Ethical Indications

For resort to high-tech home care to be ethically justified, a number of important conditions must be met. First and foremost, the decision must be "indicated" both medically and ethically. By this we mean that the proposed high-tech regimen should be not only feasible from a purely technical point of view but also justified according to a calculus of benefit and burden. Patients who would only stand to be significantly burdened by the imposition of high-tech procedures at home should not be subjected to them. This is an obvious and minimal standard, an instance of the reliable maxim that if something is not worth doing, it is not worth doing at home.

At this early stage of the process, those responsible for the patient's discharge to home should also be alert to the existence of possible psychological, social, or cultural barriers to effective care. A patient may be too proud to accept care from a spouse or daughter. A husband who is supposed to deliver care may also be untrustworthy or alcoholic. A home in a blighted neighborhood may lack adequate electrical facilities, a refrigerator, phone, or minimal sanitation. Every patient's discharge plan should be sensitive to such important factors so that they might be mitigated, when feasible, through additional psychosocial supports. When such additional support is unlikely to be forthcoming, high-tech home care may not be an appropriate alternative for the patient.

Instead of warily approaching such decisions with a fear of being overly burdened, it is our impression and that of many clinicians that most family members and close friends genuinely want to do what they can to facilitate a loved one's return home. So long as our society values this kind of home care, it should, through its medical professionals and home care specialists, enable family and friends to undertake this strenuous kind of caring (see chap. 9, this volume). This would necessarily entail adequate education for both patients and caregivers in the use of high-tech medical devices, and their implications for living and dying, *before* the patient goes home. It would also include reasonable access to personnel who could undertake on behalf of caregivers the arcane and onerous tasks of assembling a reasonable "package" of services, including the devices themselves, drugs, and ongoing supportive and supervisory personnel. Individuals like Mr. Chao, who are already experiencing tremendous stress, should not be forced to shop on the open medical market for services whose nature and monetary value they do not understand.

Communication and Consent

In addition to being "medically indicated," decisions to send a patient home on high-tech devices must satisfy the usual canons of genuinely informed consent. In the first place, the decision by a patient to accept high-tech home care—or of family and friends to care for the patient at home—must be adequately informed. This means that during the discharge-planning process at the hospital, physicians, nurses, social workers, and others should engage prospective patients and caregivers in a meaningful series of conversations bearing on the likely benefits and burdens of high-tech home care. In addition to the obvious and important benefits, caregivers need to understand fully what high-tech home care involves before their eventual consent can be said to be adequately informed. They must know, for instance, about the kinds of technical challenges they face, the likely stresses and strains of providing care, the likelihood of having to forgo work and other pursuits outside the home, the impact of visiting technicians and caregivers on family privacy, the out-of-pocket costs of high-tech home care, and so on. This is not to say, of course, that the informed consent discussion should dwell disproportionately on the possible or likely burdens of caregiving; rather, it should be a well-balanced presentation of *both* benefits and burdens.

Finally, in conformity with the ethics and law of informed consent in other settings, patients and their families should be fully apprised of the alternatives to home care, assuming that any exist and are reasonably accessible, even if such options are economically undesirable for the hospital. As we shall see presently, the absence of meaningful alternatives to high-tech home care in most communities is a major policy problem with serious implications for individual patients and families.

Justice within Caring: Limits of Familial and Friendship-Based Duties

Although society should, within the limits of reasonable health care and social services budgets, first attempt to enable families and close friends to provide desired and needed high-tech home care to loved ones, we must also begin to recognize and take seriously the limits of what can or should be expected from home caregivers. And although we are naturally reluctant to interject the public concepts and vocabulary of justice into the private sanctuary of home, a space where talk of rights often seems out of place, we must acknowledge that an ethic of care must be supplemented by a concern for the personhood of the caregivers, a concern that expresses itself in the language of "just caring" (Carse 1993).

Although a single-minded concern to advance the wishes and well-being of the patient might be justifiable within the acute care setting—where the interests of the patient in autonomy and bodily integrity usually outweigh the competing interests of others, and where life and death often hang in the balance—it is manifestly inappropriate in the home care setting. Most decisions about care in the home concern the issue of how to live, not whether to live, and these decisions usually implicate the real and weighty interests of persons other than the patient, persons whose lives, careers, and emotional balance may be drastically upset by a decision to participate in a home care plan. Thus, the systematic exclusion of the interests of family and friends who provide care at home is untenable and unjust. As technology is transferred from hospital to home, we cannot ignore the burdens this sometimes places on caregivers in the name of patient autonomy or "best interests." We must recognize that others besides the patient have legitimate needs and claims and that the resulting conflict should not always be resolved in favor of the patient.

In the context of home, where placement and treatment decisions can have enormous impact on the lives of caring friends and family, conflicting interests must be mediated and sometimes resolved in favor of these others, not dismissed out of hand, as they tend to be in hospital settings.

Although it is neither possible nor desirable to fix some kind of abstract outer boundary either to an ethic of care or to more traditional notions of familial duty, the reason for setting such limits in concrete situations is simple and compelling: the same family and friends who administer high-tech care at home are people too. Sometimes the task of mastering the technologies proves too much for certain caregivers, who end up living in a constant and seemingly endless state of panic and dread. For many others, however, the problem isn't merely technical in this narrow sense. They may have mastered the techniques but find that their entire lives have been reduced to caring for the patient and tending the machines. The demands of high-tech home care have effectively precluded any possibility of employment or meaningful social intercourse outside the home. For poor women with children on ventilators, for example, this often means that they must stay on public assistance rather than achieving some measure of dignified independence through a job outside the home.

We contend that any ethic of care or more standard account of familial duty that demands the suppression of an individual's own point of view—that negates the importance of her own projects, values, aspirations, and, in effect, her personhood—must be rejected as unjust. This kind of injustice actually operates on two distinct levels. In addition to the level of the individual case, where the abstract and ungendered language of "personhood" might suffice, there is also the historical or social dimension, in which the burdens of this erosion of personhood tend to fall disproportionately on women. This second level, often neglected in discussions of home care, amounts to a kind of institutionalized, gender-based discrimination. In morally analyzing the phenomenon of high-tech home care, then, we must be attentive not merely to the injustices embedded in the individual case but also to structural inequities pervasive of both the private and the public spheres.

Many women in the so-called sandwich generation find themselves having to divide all their time and energy between their elderly parents and their children. Moreover, many of the women providing care to elderly parents are themselves elderly. In their seventies, they take care of their "old old" parents, albeit with diminished energy, depleted funds, and mounting physical disabilities. Should a woman be tempted to refuse cooperation with a high-tech home care discharge plan, she may be consumed with guilt. The forces arrayed on the other side are powerful and motivated by self-interest. High-tech companies are concerned with profit, while hospitals stand to save money from early discharge to the home; neither can be trusted to give a well-balanced presentation of the benefits and burdens of the proposed plan to the likely caregivers. Indeed, with few exceptions, the relevant professional guidelines and norms do not even suggest, let alone require, that relating to the family in an even-handed manner is their ethical and professional obligation. The notion that involved caregivers have substantial concerns and interests that may lead them morally to refuse to cooperate in a high-tech home care plan is rarely mentioned to the family.

Where the line should be drawn, however, between reasonable impulses and duties to care, on the one hand, and unconscionable demands, on the other, will always be a difficult and anxiety-ridden judgment call. Given the complexity of the home care setting, the wide spectrum of benefits and burdens imparted by various technologies, and the tangled histories of families and their individual members, no general rule will suffice. The details of personal histories and relationships must be taken into account. Perhaps a devoted son cannot change the soiled diapers of his mother, a formerly abused daughter should not be asked to take her abusing father into her home, or the parents of a technology-dependent child suddenly realize that the demands of caring have begun to eclipse their own lives and the lives of their other children. In every case, the limits of caring will be discernable only against the backdrop of a particular narrative of family relationships, the type and duration of care, and the particular objectives of the treatment.

None of this talk of unjust burden-dumping is meant to suggest the impossibility of certain highly dedicated people wishing to shoulder such all-encompassing burdens of their own accord. Motivated, perhaps, by a spirit of altruism, community, filial love, or religiously inspired self-sacrifice, some individuals may freely choose such a course of hardship and self-abnegation. While we have no problem with particular individuals, usually women, *freely choosing* such a life plan, we would insist on the deeply compromised and problematic circumstances of most such choices. Against the backdrop of strong societal expectations for women to conform to stereotypical roles (e.g., the devoted, caring wife, mother, daughter) and the absence of viable alternatives for equally loving care either in or outside the home, a "free choice" to subordinate oneself totally to the care of another begins to look increasingly problematic, increasingly unfree. These observations about just caring suggest that the *accommodation* (Dubler 1990) and *mediation* (Dubler and Marcus 1994) of all legitimate interests, rather than the exclusionary pursuit of the patient's autonomy or best interests, are the most appropriate models for thinking about the justice of interpersonal relationships within high-tech home care. Those who provide loving care, tend the machines, administer the medications, deal with the vendors, change the diapers, and put their lives on hold have serious interests that must be taken into account in any *just* home care plan. When their legitimate interests conflict with the interests of patients, our first response should be to find some mutually acceptable accommodation or compromise, preferably through informal channels of mediation. In case a smooth, mutually agreeable accommodation cannot be reached, we see no reason why caregivers threatened with the near-extinction of their personal lives must always be sacrificed to the desires or best interests of the patient.

The fact that there are limits to what might reasonably be expected from caregivers means that some families with limited financial, physical, or emotional resources might ethically refuse to undertake the home care of a technologically dependent patient (or indeed of any especially burdensome patient). In a just society that insisted on the continuing care and treatment of such patients, families would not be pressured or made to feel guilty for wishing to avoid what they reasonably anticipate to be an unsupportable burden. The fact of moral limits likewise means that even after family or friends have undertaken the high-tech care of a patient at home, they should reserve the right to change their minds, without being subjected to moral opprobrium, should the burdens eventually become too great. Indeed, patients should be counseled at the outset that all arrangements are on a trial basis and will be periodically reevaluated. As many commentators have noted with regard to the alleged moral distinction between withdrawing and withholding medical treatments, the same reasons that provide a warrant for not starting should also apply to stopping something already begun. Also, if we think it in general a good idea that families consent to a trial of treatment, whether it be life-sustaining measures in a hospital or high-tech home care, rather than precipitously declining options that *might* work, then it is crucial to offer them this kind of moral "escape hatch." Otherwise, families and caregivers will be reluctant to start something worthwhile for fear that they might not be able to finish. Treatment contracts for high-tech home care should thus be not only based on genuinely informed consent but also explicitly renegotiable throughout the course of the patient's care.

Alternative Institutions

The emotional resonance of "home" is so great in our culture that there is a tendency to romanticize the home setting in discussions of high-tech home care. Many people tend to think that the worst home is better than the best hospital or long-term care facility, but this is not necessarily so. As we have already seen, the rigors of high-tech home care can overwhelm and transform some homes to the point that there remains nothing "homelike" about them. Caregivers can be overburdened and patients themselves can occasionally be misplaced at home, where fear of pain and technological failure can come to dominate their lives. Although many, perhaps most, patients keenly prefer their home to the hospital, home care might sometimes pose larger threats to autonomy and privacy than well-designed alternative institutions whose staff would always be available but perhaps not as intrusive as family members. Patients with overbearing families or those who do not wish to impose the burdens of high-tech home care on their loved ones might well prefer some other setting.

While such reflections certainly do not argue for a wholesale repudiation of high-tech home care, they should make us skeptical of any headlong societal embrace of the home as the universal solution. Instead of pushing everyone with high-tech requirements into home care, we should consider the alternative of creating and sustaining a variety of institutions that might better serve certain categories of patients and their families. Indeed, the home may look so good to us now precisely because the alternatives, including nursing homes and other long-term care facilities, look so bad. Apart from upgrading existing institutions and providing more respite care to beleaguered families, we should also investigate the possibility and wisdom of establishing new institutional structures intermediate between hospital and home. Instead of channeling this new technology into established but often inappropriate structures, we might envision a different kind of institution: for example, a small-scale, residential facility capable of providing all the necessary technical support for high-tech care while looking and feeling more like a home than a miniature intensive care unit or nursing home.

Indeed, we would argue that the establishment of such meaning-ful alternatives to home care for patients with high-tech needs is a prerequisite for genuine and sustained consent to high-tech home care. To be valid, consent must not only be informed but also freely given. But many patients and families, lacking any decent alternatives between hospital and home, are presently forced to opt for home care even when it is likely to have a devastating impact on their home life and finances. Likewise, it is impossible to insist that home care "contracts" should be continuously revisable, that patients and families should be able to opt out when the stresses become unsupportable, in the absence of viable alternatives. Unless families have access to such alternatives, their initial acceptance of the home care plan becomes a trap from which there is no practical escape. We thus begin to see how a moral assessment of individual high-tech home care arrangements requires certain preconditions on the level of social policy.

Mapping the Policy Dimensions of High-Tech Home Care

The boom in the market for high-tech home care has been spectacular, featuring an overall rate of growth of about 20 to 25 percent per year (Feder 1991; Spiegel 1991; chap. 13, below). For-profit companies have proliferated and prospered in an atmosphere reminiscent of the Wild West. Since relatively little public money has been devoted to high-tech home care until quite recently, and since most of this care has been paid for either by private insurance companies or out of pocket, Congress has been slow to pay heed to this phenomenon and to acknowledge its excesses and abuses. Largely unfettered and even unnoticed by regulators, vendor companies have taken full advantage of this leeway and amassed enormous profits through questionable sales practices and astonishing price markups.

One such questionable sales practice involves the marketing of high-tech devices directly to patients at home. Always on the lookout for ways to expand their penetration of the market, some vendors of high-tech instruments and services have attempted to contact patients directly, often by phone, and sell them expensive hardware that may not even be relevant to their medical condition. Vendors have also attempted to obtain information about specific patients from hospital outpatient clinics and then importune the patients' physicians with certificates of medical necessity, which some harried and distracted physicians have signed (Pear 1991). Although some of these devices, such as TENS units (transcutaneous electrical nerve stimulators), can benefit some patients, most merely gather dust when sold in this fashion directly to patients, many of whom are elderly and easy prey to unscrupulous entrepreneurs.

Even more dramatic is the extent of price gouging in the high-tech home care industry. According to Mark Green, New York City's former commissioner of consumer affairs, abuses in the high-tech home care market for AIDS patients are particularly disturbing (City of New York DCA 1991). Green's report documented some egregious examples of overcharging by high-tech companies: a 10-ml bottle of sterile water, available for $2.00 at a pharmacy, cost some consumers $9.84; a $4.00 pharmacy-prepared dextrose solution can cost $22.22; and various home care equipment items, whose unit cost may be 15 or 20 cents, have been billed at or around $35—amounting to mark-ups of 2000 to 3000 percent.

From the viewpoint of health policy, however, by far the most important and disturbing example is the cost of TPN for AIDS care. Again according to Green's report, the market for TPN, which reached $622 million in 1991, accounts for 21 percent of the total home infusion market. With nearly half of all AIDS patients eventually receiving TPN, this treatment accounts for roughly one-third of the estimated $150,000 average lifetime cost of caring for an individual with AIDS. In Green's study, the average reported cost of TPN was $377 per day, which added up to more than $10,000 per month and culminated, after the addition of related charges, in charges approaching $16,000. According to Green's office, a realistic charge, based on actual costs, would look more like $1,300 per month.

Almost as disturbing as the cost of these services is the reluctance of high-tech home care vendors to disclose their actual costs or prices, making public oversight, comparison shopping, or the establishment of fee schedules almost impossible. Only three of twelve companies responded to Green's persistent requests for information.

The result of this secrecy and overcharging is a market in high-tech home care that is enormously profitable but responsible for highly inflated charges that often bear no relationship to actual costs that most likely rival or even outstrip the cost of in-patient hospital care for AIDS patients. The relative cost advantage of home over hospital care is even more doubtful when we factor in the serious opportunity costs of high-tech home care for families. As we noted above, family caregivers responsible for high-tech services usually have to forgo the possibility of employment outside the home. Given the increasing amounts of public money for high-tech home care paid by the federal government and the growing skepticism of insurance companies, increased regulation is both necessary and inevitable.

Whether high-tech home care is more cost-effective than comparable care in institutions is a complicated and difficult question to answer (chap. 13, this volume). Given the wide variety of high-tech interventions, it is likely that some will be more cost-effective in the home, while others will be less costly if administered in hospitals. Still, if our experience with garden-variety home care is a reliable indicator, we should not expect to reap substantial savings overall from deploying high-tech care in the home. A coordinated evaluation of twenty-seven studies conducted in ten states demonstrated conclusively that (ordinary) home care led to increased spending, failed to provide positive benefits in terms of longevity and mental functioning, and increased the risk of clients' physical dependence on caretakers, compared with similar populations in long-term care facilities. Researchers could demonstrate the superiority of home to institutional care only in enhancing clients' sense of contentment (or "life satisfaction"), and even this positive advantage was relatively small and tended to dissipate after a year (Weissert 1991).

On the basis of this experience, it would not be implausible to predict that new high-tech home care ventures will be equally driven by patient demand as well as by hospitals' cost consciousness and the industry's desire for profits. None of these driving forces, including patient demand, constitutes an adequate basis for public policy regarding the dissemination of high-tech home care. Instead of more sporadic and ad hoc attempts to deliver new high-tech services to new categories of patients, attempts that we would describe as unsupervised and unevaluated clinical trials, we need to identify and measure those factors that might support rational and coherent pubic policy discussions in this area.

Another troubling feature of the unrestrained profit-driven market in high-tech home care is the high degree of specialization among vendors. Before the rise of high technology, nurses delivering home care tended to view the patient from a holistic perspective, in accordance with the generalist ethos of their profession. Many high-tech home care companies, by contrast, market a service, but make their profits selling devices, drugs, and intravenous fluids. As a result, the care provided by these companies often tends to be narrowly focused on servicing technologies, sometimes to the point of overlooking symptoms unrelated, for example, to the upkeep of an infusion pump. In addition, such a high degree of specialization among "boutique agencies" and their service personnel can frequently lead to fragmented, depersonalized, and uncoordinated care, precisely the kind of service that we tend to associate with hospitals rather than home. For many home-bound patients, "high tech" can thus be an unsatisfactory substitute for "high touch."

A Skeptical Challenge

An observer contemplating the scene we have sketched in this chapter could not be blamed for harboring serious reservations about the entire high-tech home care enterprise. Echoing themes from Daniel Callahan's work (1987, 1991), she might claim that in an era of belt-tightening in medicine, at a time when we need to shift our priorities for vast numbers of patients away from costly yet marginally curative measures toward an ethos of low-tech caring, the last thing we need is a whole new category of high-tech, high-cost, high-profit services of highly questionable efficacy. "This kind of 'caring,' " she might object, "is nothing more than a capitalistic parody of the kind of low-tech, caring system that we need for our dying AIDS and cancer patients, impaired elderly persons, and severely afflicted newborns—a parody in which caring has been transformed into a depersonalized, high-tech business."

Although such a broad-gauged critique assumes an initial plausibility when viewed against the backdrop of the inefficiencies, excesses, and injustices of the high-tech home care industry, it is far too sweeping in scope to serve as a guide to policy. As Norman Daniels argues in chapter 14, below, some essential preconditions of ethically acceptable rationing are missing from this debate. We have no fair, public, democratic procedure for deciding whether and how to ration or eliminate high-tech home services; we have no closed, global health care budget that would allow us to argue justifiably that money saved on services of dubious value would be put to better use elsewhere in the system; and, perhaps most important, we lack reliable information about the costs and benefits not only of high-tech services but also of many hospital- or institution-based alternative services. In the absence of democratic procedures, global budgeting, and comparative efficacy data, we are not in a good position to make sweeping denunciations of the entire high-tech home care enterprise.

To be sure, each of the above deficiencies could be remedied. We could, for example, follow Oregon's example by creating democratically appointed and accountable health services commissions in every state—and perhaps also on the federal level—that would be charged with the tasks of technology assessment and priority setting. We could also impose global limits on health care spending, limits that might allow us to weigh the benefits and costs, including opportunity costs, of competing technologies and services within a systematic budget. Even were we to accomplish all this, however, it is not clear that high-tech home care services would be a ripe candidate for categorical rationing, as the skeptical challenge asserts.

This is because the data, once finally in hand, would reveal a vast spectrum of high-tech interventions, some of which will be proven to be relatively effective, inexpensive, and "caregiver friendly" vis-à-vis the alternatives, and which should accordingly be included in any reasonable package of health care benefits and services. Plausible examples might be high-tech pain-control devices for dying, homebound cancer patients or TPN for AIDS patients with severe diarrhea. To be sure, such studies will also show that some of our current practices are only marginally, if at all, effective and much too expensive, at least at current prices, to be offered routinely to patients or reimbursed by health plans and insurers. A possible example here might be the routine deployment of TPN for end-stage AIDS patients presenting, not with diarrhea but with severe anorexia, at a cost of $15,000 per month. The basic point, however, is that the crucial factors bearing on allocation or rationing decisions of high-tech home care will have to do with traditional indicia of cost and effectiveness, benefits and burdens (to both patients and families), opportunity costs for other patients and services, and the impact of treatments on such philosophically relevant variables as patient welfare, equality of opportunity, and community solidarity. Whether a proposed form of treatment is high tech or low tech is, in itself, a morally irrelevant distinction vis-à-vis the allocation question.

The Place of High-Tech Home Care in the Health Care System

A serious and responsible debate about the place of high-tech home care within our overall "system" of health care will have to await the fulfillment of Daniels's above-mentioned criteria for just allocations of health care. There will have to be an accountable public agency, a closed system in which the full costs and benefits of alternative treatments and sites of care can be meaningfully compared, and, perhaps most important, we will need reliable data on those costs and benefits, data that we presently lack. We can, however, presently attempt to formulate some important questions for that future debate.

One crucial question concerns the establishment of priorities among medical and nonmedical services—such as help with cooking, cleaning, bathing, dressings, and other basic personal and safety needs—that enhance the quality of life for the homebound and effectively keep many individuals out of the hospital in the first place. Although we argued above that the bare difference between high tech and low tech does not necessarily mark an important difference for public policy purposes, it nevertheless strikes us as highly anomalous that hundreds of millions, if not billions, of dollars are currently being poured into high-tech home care when the basic needs of many patients for nonmedical community supports often go unmet. This criticism supports the agenda of disabilities groups for increased access to community-based support services for people unable to perform important tasks of daily living (Litvak, Zukas, and Heumann 1987). While such services lack the glamour and profitability of the more medicalized sectors of home care, studies have shown that, at least in the elderly population, supportive, high-touch care is most needed by people living at home with chronic illnesses and functional difficulties (Jones, Densen, and Brown 1989).

In the context of our present, competitive, market-oriented nonsystem of health care delivery, money clearly drives health policy. Instead of wisely investing money, for example, in relatively cheap prenatal care and nutrition for pregnant women, our society prefers to spend millions on high-tech neonatal nurseries that attend to the inevitable and costly sequelae of low birthweight. In the area of home care, high tech is clearly where the money is. But whether most high-tech home care interventions would claim pride of place in a reformed health care system that stressed the universal satisfaction of basic needs and primary care is a very open question, one that deserves careful scrutiny in future debates about health policy.

A Public Policy Agenda

In view of the numerous policy-level problems this project has highlighted—including overcharging, inappropriate marketing, the absence of standards and data regarding safety, efficacy, and quality—closer supervision of the high-tech home care industry is clearly desirable and necessary. To be sure, market forces are already beginning to erode the industry's ability to charge insurers and individuals whatever it wishes, but we doubt that the market alone can be relied on adequately to protect the vital interests of patients and their families. We suggest, then, that the following steps be taken toward the reform of high-tech home care policy.

We recommend that one or more congressional committees concerned with health, aging, and care for persons with disabilities hold hearings to gather much-needed data on high-tech home care. Perhaps the greatest need in the area of social policy is for reliable information and carefully wrought standards regarding costs, reimbursement practices, quality, access, case management, family support, and feasible alternatives to high-tech home care. Once these congressional investigations have focused the nation's attention on the nature and scope of these problems, private research groups and other organs of government—such as the Health Care Financing Administration and the Agency for Health Care Policy and Research—might then undertake well-targeted research projects to provide the missing data and, in conjunction with professional and consumer organizations, appropriate standards for evaluation.

State departments of health are already in the business of regulating long-term care, including home care, and we recommend that they extend the ambit of their regulatory activities to include high-tech home care. In addition to tracking the above federal efforts, state agencies should begin to conduct their own research and to amass their own data on the phenomenon of high-tech home care. Once they have gathered sufficient information from professional, consumer, and industry sources, states should require the establishment of measures for evaluating the quality, safety, effectiveness, and cost of high-tech home interventions in general and as applied to particular categories of patients.

Apart from gathering information and forging standards, however, we contend that states already know enough to require that all high-tech home care agencies file annual reports detailing the actual cost of their services, the prices charged to consumers, and any special rates provided for various individuals or groups. In addition, states should require for every high-tech home care patient a comprehensive plan of care, including a discussion of the benefits and burdens of such care with patients and their families, options for family support, and the provision of case management.

Conclusion

Notwithstanding their manifest importance, abstract discussions of risks, costs, and equity do not capture the compelling human dimensions of high-tech home care. We were deeply moved by the stories of those family members, friends, and health care professionals who have begun to inhabit this brave new world full of hope and peril. The narratives of Mrs. Borrero, Mr. Chao, and others helped us understand the importance to the caregivers of being given the opportunity to care. This benefit was as important for them as it was for their patients. To be sure, all the caregivers experienced some ambivalence about the demanding and unending nature of the role, but all shouldered the burdens with relative good humor and an appreciation of the special meaning of the experience for their own identities and their relationships with loved ones.

High-tech home care thus simultaneously provides the opportunity for love and the means of exploitation. To maximize the former and minimize the latter, we must begin to think more critically about the phenomenon of high-tech home care. Instead of allowing this technology to develop of its own internal dynamics or, worse, according to the dictates of the profit motive, we must begin to ask how high-tech home care might best serve human needs and the needs of a compassionate but prudent society.

REFERENCES

American Medical Association (AMA), Council on Scientific Affairs. 1991. Educating physicians in home health care. *JAMA* 265:769.

Arras, J. D. 1995. Conflicting interests in long-term care. In N. Wilson and L. McCullough, eds., *Long-Term Care Decisions: Ethical and Conceptual Dimensions*. Baltimore: Johns Hopkins University Press.

Callahan, D. 1987. *Setting Limits*. New York: Simon and Schuster.

———. 1991. *What Kind of Life?* New York: Simon and Schuster.

Carse, A. L. 1993. Justice within intimate spheres. *Journal of Clinical Ethics* 4:68–71.

City of New York, Department of Consumer Affairs (DCA). 1991. *Making a Killing on AIDS: Home Health Care and Pentamidine*, (May).

Corbin, J. M., and Strauss, A.L. 1988. *Unending Work and Care: Managing Chronic Illness at Home*. San Francisco: Jossey-Bass.

Dubler, N. N. 1990. Accommodating the home care client. In C. Zuckerman, N. N. Dubler, and B. Collopy, eds., *Home Health Care Options: A Guide for Older Persons and Concerned Families*, pp. 141–65. New York: Plenum Press.

Dubler, N. N., and Marcus, L. 1994. *Mediating Bioethical Disputes: A Practical Guide*. New York: United Hospital Fund of New York.

Ellul, J. 1964. *The Technological Society* New York: Knopf.

Feder, B. J. 1991. Where the boom is in health care. *New York Times*, 26 December.

Goldberg, A. I. 1983. *Home Care Services for Severely Physically Disabled People in England and France*. Washington, D.C.: National Institute of Handicapped Research, U.S. Department of Education.

Illich, I. 1976. *Medical Nemesis: The Expropriation of Health*. New York: Pantheon.

Jones, E. W., Densen, P. M., and Brown, S. D. 1989. Posthospital needs of elderly people at home. *Health Services Research* 24:643–63.

Kane, R. A., and Reinardy, J. 1990. Family caregiving in home care. In C. Zuckerman, N. N. Dubler, and B. Collopy, eds., *Home Health Care Options: A Guide for Older Persons and Concerned Families*, pp. 89–113. New York: Plenum Press.

Kohrman, A. F. 1991. Psychological issues. In M. J. Mehlman and S. J. Youngner, eds., *Delivering High Technology Home Care*, pp. 168–69. New York: Springer.

Lantos, J. D., and Kohrman, A. F. 1992. Ethical aspects of pediatric home care. *Pediatrics* 89:920–24.

Larkin, H. 1992. High-tech home care dilemma: Physicians face payment struggle to get patients out of the hospital. *AMA News*, 8 June, p. 9.

Litvak, S., Zukas, H., and Heumann, J. 1987. *Attending to America: Personal Assistance for Independent Living.* Berkeley: World Institute on Disability.

Monette, P. 1988. *Borrowed Time: An AIDS Memoir.* New York: Avon Books.

Pear, R. 1991. Abuse widespread in medical sales for care at home. *New York Times* 29 September.

Rhoden, N. 1988. Litigating life and death. *Harvard Law Review* 102:425–29.

Siwek, J. 1989. House calls: current status and rationale. *American Family Physician* 31:169–74.

Spiegel, A. D. 1991. The economics of high-technology home care: doing right for the wrong reason. In M. J. Mehlman and S. J. Youngner, eds., *Delivering High Technology Home Care*, pp. 23–66. New York: Springer.

van den Boom, F. 1991. AIDS in the family: a personal reflection. *AIDS Patient Care*, December, pp. 273–79.

Weissert, W.G. 1991. A new policy agenda for home care. *Health Affairs* 1:68.

Winner, L. 1977. *Autonomous technology: technics-out-of-control as a theme in political thought.* Cambridge, Mass.: M.I.T. University Press.

I. The Technologies and Their Effects on Patients and Families

2. The History of Respirators and Total Parenteral Nutrition in the Home and Their Use in Children Today

Alex Okun, M.D.

Many people outside the health care or teaching professions find it hard to imagine a boisterous child tethered to a ventilator or feeding pump in the home. Most picture "technology-dependent children" as frail, premature babies taped to tubes and wires in intensive care units. Yet thousands of children at home today lead lives considered to be safe, predictable, and fulfilling with high-technology equipment at their side.

This chapter on home care for children focuses on two technologies on which most of these children's lives depend: mechanical respirators and total parenteral nutrition (TPN). The invention and development of these technologies is reviewed. The history of their use in children's homes is explored in detail, with the aim of understanding for whom these technologies work out well and at what costs.

Mechanical Respirators: Efficacy and Risks

A mechanical respirator, also called a ventilator, is a machine that forces air into the lungs. It is used when the muscles of breathing or the lungs themselves cannot provide an adequate supply of oxygen or remove enough carbon dioxide waste. In this chapter, the terms "respirator" and "ventilator" are used interchangeably.

A negative-pressure respirator works by creating a vacuum inside a tank or body jacket that encases someone from the neck down. As the vacuum increases, the chest expands and air is drawn in through the mouth and nose. In 1889, Alexander Graham Bell designed and built the first such respirator for newborns, consisting of a chest jacket and hand-operated bellows. He wrote: "Many children, especially those prematurely born, die from an inability to expand their lungs sufficiently when they take their first breath. I have no doubt that in many of those cases, lives could be saved by starting the respiration artificially by means of an apparatus operating in the manner [described above]" (Stern et al. 1970, p. 595). The results of animal studies presented by Bell to the American Association for the Advancement of Science met with little enthusiasm. Nearly forty years later, an 8-year-old girl with respiratory failure from poliomyelitis became the first patient to be supported for days on a negative-pressure respirator (Drinker and Shaw 1929) powered entirely by electricity (Markel 1994).

A positive-pressure respirator, in contrast, pumps air directly into a tube connected to someone's trachea. First used in the 1920s for operative patients under anesthesia (Cane and Shapiro 1985), it later became the preferred method to ventilate conscious patients by providing better access to the body and airway and superior movement of stiff lungs (Engstrom 1963; Lassen 1953; Snider 1989). (The workings of respirators are described further in chap. 7, below.)

Positive-pressure respirators include alarms to signal when the person is disconnected from the machine or when some point between the machine and the person's lungs is obstructed. It is possible to control the temperature, humidity, and oxygen content of the air, as well as the frequency, force, rapidity, and timing with which breaths are delivered by the machine. Although most hospital units are the size of a small refrigerator, some positive-pressure respirators are designed to be portable, fitting on the back of a wheelchair or in a child's "little red wagon" along with the necessary battery, oxygen tank, suction machine, and supplies.

A child may need mechanical ventilation for any of several reasons. In the case of central hypoventilation, the brain, during sleep, fails to signal the breathing apparatus enough or at all. In children with high spinal cord lesions due to trauma, inflammatory disorders, polio, or other infections, the brain is not able to transmit the signal to breathe down the spinal cord to the muscles of the chest and diaphragm. Some children with advanced neuromuscular disease are too weak to breathe deeply or often enough to survive without mechanical ventilation. In advanced intrinsic pulmonary disorders, the lungs are stiff and take up oxygen poorly. Many anatomic abnormalities of the airway can be overcome by the ability of the positive-pressure respirator to tent open an obstruction or bypass the problem entirely. Mechanical ventilation can permit survival in these situations, used intermittently or throughout the day.

During the polio epidemics of the 1940s and 1950s in the United States, negative-pressure ventilators were used widely in respiratory rehabilitation programs established under the auspices of the National Foundation for Infantile Paralysis, or the March of Dimes (Goldberg 1992). Harrison and Mitchell (1961) described the course of 200 patients, many of them children, an average of eleven years after admission to the Southwestern Poliomyelitis Respiratory and Rehabilitation Center. One-third were off all ventilatory support at follow-up.

The success with polio patients encouraged the application of negative-pressure respirators to patients at home with other debilitating neuromuscular conditions. Children with muscular dystrophy lived longer than anticipated (Alexander et al. 1979) as carbon dioxide retention and pulmonary hypertension improved (O'Leary et al., 1979).

Once infants with tracheostomies were considered safe to discharge from hospitals (Foster and Hoskins 1981; Ruben et al. 1982), positive-pressure respirators, which connect to tracheostomy tubes, began being used for young children in the home. In the late 1970s, an innovative home ventilator program was developed in Philadelphia specifically for survivors of neonatal and pediatric intensive care. Complications and morbidity were low (Goldberg et al. 1980).

At other centers, use of respirators in the home was accompanied by some serious risks and disappointments. Alcock et al. (1984) followed 113 ventilator-dependent polio survivors at home in and around Manitoba for over twenty years. While 19 percent of the patients felt that their level of respiratory impairment had improved, 56 percent felt it was the same, and 27 percent felt it was worse than it had been a year after they returned home. Among 47 ventilator-dependent children and adults from Houston with spinal cord injury, neuromuscular disease, or cardiorespiratory conditions, half of those under 11 years of age (9 of 18) died in their first three years at home (Splaingard et al. 1983). Two died by disconnection from the ventilator and two for unknown reasons, prompting the authors and others to call for better monitors and alarms (Frates, Harrison, and Splaingard 1984; Goldberg 1983;).

Home care for ventilator-dependent children in the United States was largely privately funded by families or their insurance companies until 1981. The care of many children has since been subsidized publicly through legislation that began with President Ronald Reagan's approval of the Katie Beckett Waiver. This allowed Medicaid funding for the home care of a 5-year-old girl from Iowa, ventilator-dependent after encephalitis, who remained hospitalized because of her family's inability to afford care for her at home. That same year, the Health Care Financing Administration approved the Medicaid Home and Community-Based Services Waiver Program. This assured funding in each state for the home care of fifty technology-dependent children and an additional fifty blind or disabled children and adults who, in the absence of community services, would otherwise require long-term institutional care.

Six years later, based on estimates from state programs, national data sets, and commercial registries, the U.S. Congress Office of Technology Assessment (OTA) (1987) projected that 680 to 2000 children were living at home on mechanical respirators all or part of their day. Forty-one were counted in Massachusetts alone (Palfrey et al. 1991).

Ventilator-dependent children can expect to live for years at home. Sadly, respirators do nothing to cure the underlying conditions that mandate their use. Children can die or suffer severe damage from machine failure, airway obstruction, or progression of their disease. Respirators are highly effective in the home, but at substantial risk.

Total Parenteral Nutrition: Efficacy and Risks

TPN is a liquid mixture pumped directly into the bloodstream, providing all nutrients necessary for growth and healing. This balanced intravenous diet contains water, sugar, electrolytes, vitamins, minerals, trace elements, fats, and proteins or amino acids.

Children receive TPN in the home for any of several conditions. In some, the intestines are severely damaged because of radiation, infection, or inflammatory disease and may require prolonged rest without feeding in order to heal. In others, the intestines may lack sufficient absorptive surface because of congenital malformation, trauma or surgery. In those with severe motility disorders, the food is not moved along the intestines properly. Some children in hypermetabolic states due to cancer or AIDS cannot take in sufficient nutrition by mouth to meet their enormous caloric needs. (Indications for TPN in cancer patients and in elderly persons are identified, respectively, in chaps. 4 and 7, below.)

In 1987, the U.S. Congress Office of Technology Assessment estimated that 350 to 750 children were home on TPN (OTA 1987). That year in Massachusetts, 158 children were dependent on intravenous feeding devices in the home (Palfrey et al. 1991), nearly half on TPN.

The era of TPN had begun fifty years earlier (Heird 1987). Protein hydrolysates infused in hospitalized patients in the 1930s provided some improvement in nutritional status, but weight gain was achieved only after cottonseed oil or glucose was added to the intravenous solution. The first case of positive nitrogen balance and weight gain in a child on exclusive intravenous feeding was a 5-month-old with malnutrition due to a severe motility disorder, fed for five days with alternating infusions of 50 percent glucose, 10 percent casein hydrolysate, and olive oil–lecithin emulsions (Helfrick and Abelson, 1944). By the end of this period, "the fat pads of the cheek had returned, the ribs were less prominent, and the general nutritional status was much improved. His former expression of dire misery was gone" (p. 402).

After successful trials in beagle puppies, Dudrick et al. (1968) produced normal growth in a four-pound infant born with multiple atresias of the small intestine by infusing TPN into a central vein. The use of a large vein was necessary because glucose infusions concentrated enough to provide weight gain destroyed peripheral veins accessible by conventional catheters.

Normal growth and nutritional rehabilitation were soon reported in a series of hospitalized adults on central venous TPN as the sole source of nutrition (Dudrick et al. 1969). The first patient reported to receive TPN at home was a 36-year-old woman with ovarian cancer, a mother with small children, in 1969. She lived six months longer and with better quality of life than anticipated had she not been nourished with TPN (Dudrick 1981). An "artificial gut system" was soon developed by Scribner et al. (1970), in which TPN was infused at home for twelve to eighteen hours a day. This permitted greater freedom than the continuous regimen prescribed in hospitals until that point. Adults living at home with short bowel syndrome, chronic diarrhea, or other disorders gained weight and improved their tolerance for exercise and general sense of well-being.

In what is probably the most significant technical advance in TPN, Broviac et al. (1973) invented a Silastic, cuffed catheter that could be tunneled subcutaneously from a point beneath the clavicle or behind the ear into the superior vena cava. This catheter was less brittle than its polyvinyl predecessors (Heird 1987) and remained fixed more securely in the skin. (A range of catheters now available, some completely subcutaneous, is described in chaps. 4 and 7, below.)

By the mid-1980s, nutritional rehabilitation and the improvement of disease symptoms had been achieved in children at home on TPN with a variety of conditions, including short-bowel syndrome and motility disorders (Byrne et al. 1977; Dorney et al. 1985; Pitt et al. 1985). Children malnourished and stunted from their bowel disease displayed "catch-up growth"; all 122 infants and children reported in home TPN programs from France and England grew at accelerated rates and established normal height and weight (Bisset et al. 1992; Goulet et al. 1991; Ricour et al. 1990).

Home TPN was tested as a means of avoiding bowel resections in some patients with inflammatory bowel disease. While it did not obviate the need for surgery in one group of patients with severe disease (Fleming, McGill, and Birkner 1977), twelve of fourteen patients in another group were spared rectal operations (Dudrick 1981) because wounds and fistulas healed and symptoms of the underlying condition improved. Strobel et al. (1979) proposed TPN as a first step toward trying to avoid surgery or at least as an adjunct to it.

Most children are eventually able to stop home TPN. Up to two-thirds of those with short bowel syndrome and more with inflammatory bowel disease can expect to be off all nutritional support after several years (Ricour et al. 1990; Vargas, Ament, and Berquist 1987; Weber, Tracy, and Connors 1991).

Broviac and Scribner (1974) and Jeejeebhoy et al. (1976) focused some of the earliest attention on the risks of long-term TPN. Signs of liver inflammation appear at some point in up to 75 percent of patients on TPN (Heird 1987) but only rarely progress to cirrhosis. Specific nutrient deficiencies are common and may be difficult to correct, as with calcium or vitamin D deficiency. Copper, zinc, essential fatty acids, selenium, and biotin are easier to replace.

Babies nourished on TPN adopt a "cushingoid" appearance, with slim arms and legs and extra fat in the cheeks and trunk and between the shoulders. Intravenous fat emulsions can impair oxygen diffusion in the lungs of premature infants (Heird 1987). Small children on TPN may become anemic simply from the need to have numerous specimens of blood drawn.

Though rare, errors in the preparation or administration of TPN can be harmful or fatal. One hospitalized infant died of fluid imbalance when TPN solution was inadvertently infused into his jejunostomy rather than the catheter (Vargas, Ament, and Berquist 1987). A premature baby in intensive care died of sepsis after infant formula was accidentally administered into the TPN line (Huddleston, Creedmore, and Wood 1994).

The balance of the risks associated with home TPN is attributable to problems with the catheter. Infections around the exit site or of the subcutaneous tunnel are partly preventable with meticulous skin care. Most of these can be treated with intravenous antibiotics without removing the catheter.

Catheter sepsis, the most serious complication associated with the use of TPN, is a bacterial or fungal infection that spreads from the lumen of the catheter to the bloodstream. It occurs, on average, about once every twenty months, and roughly 1 in 200 cases in children is fatal (Decker and Edwards 1988). Cure is possible about 75 percent of the time without removing the catheter and in most of the remaining cases by taking the catheter out. Though many children keep their original catheters for years, a 2-year-old from Houston needed three replaced over eight months because of infections caused by his chewing on them (Pokorny et al. 1987).

The use of catheters is fraught with mechanical problems. Obstruction is largely preventable by the daily injection of heparin into the catheter. Fracture occurs from improper handling and clamping of the catheter, especially as it becomes more brittle with age. The catheter may become dislodged ("yanked out"), especially in active children. The tip, which normally points down the superior vena cava toward the heart, may flip up into the neck and cause circulatory symptoms. Unrecognized disconnection from the feeding solution can cause hypoglycemia and blood loss from the open end of the catheter.

TPN can nourish children long-term and, for many, bridge the period from institutionally based technological dependency to a life at home, free of pumps and catheters. Unlike the situation with ventilators, many of the underlying conditions leading to the use of TPN in the home will improve over time. As with home ventilators, this technology's gains are associated with serious, sometimes fatal risks.

The Benefits and Burdens of Respirators and TPN in the Home

One of the founders of the ventilator program for infants and children from Philadelphia, Allen Goldberg, proclaimed the home "a safe environment which promotes the health of all" (Goldberg et al. 1984). A ventilator-dependent child going home from the hospital could look forward to an improved sense of family, appropriate education, developmental interaction and stimulation from friends, and the opportunity for "spiritual growth and wellness" (Goldberg 1983). Parents from one series in Massachusetts felt confident and positive with their ventilator-dependent children at home (Burr et al. 1983).

Many children dependent on TPN are best able to meet their full potential at home (Ralston et al. 1984). The lives of some were "normalized" (Byrne et al. 1977) as they resumed activities with peer groups at school and work (Fleming, McGill, and Berkner 1977; Strobel et al. 1978). British parents found home care "rewarding and infinitely preferable" to hospitalization (Bisset et al. 1992, p. 113). Neurologic development was normal over one to three years in twenty of twenty-eight infants from Providence, Salt Lake City, and Los Angeles raised on TPN from the neonatal period (Dorney et al., 1985; Goldberger et al. 1979; Ralston et al. 1984).

The social and psychological burdens of high technology in the home were identified in the earliest reports on ventilators and TPN. Nineteen percent of polio survivors home on ventilators in Harrison and Mitchell's (1961) follow-up study experienced severe to total disruption in family integrity. The authors concluded that the "success of the home program and the extent to which the patient resumes his former role in society are based primarily on psychosocial factors rather than on the extent of the patient's physical disability and medical problem" (p. 598).

Ventilator-dependent children may have difficulty adjusting to strangers in the home (Splaingard et al. 1983). Some children raised on TPN from birth show a peculiar lack of interest in food and limited or absent appetite (Cannon et al. 1980). Five of nine older children home on TPN in Minnesota displayed more severe problems, including reclusive and separatist behavior, noncompliance, and substance abuse (Amarnath, Fleming, and Perrault 1987). In another series, young adults on TPN experienced depression, distorted body image, fear of dependence on machinery, fear of catheter manipulation, and financial hardship in their first months at home (Dwyer, Baker, and Richardson 1987).

Parents of children on ventilators in Massachusetts complained of difficult schedules, sleep disruption, limited social lives, and loss of privacy (Burr et al. 1983). Kohrman (1992) emphasized this loss of privacy and described parents' need to "hide the strains and passions of everyday life" (p. 165) from their children, other family members, and professionals. The technology-dependent child may not be the only family member with complex medical needs; three families in a Los Angeles program had more than one child home on TPN (Vargas, Ament, and Berquist 1987).

British parents who preferred home TPN to hospitalization felt trapped by the dependence of their children on the technology and found little understanding of their own needs from community agencies (Bisset et al. 1992). Kohrman (1992) wrote of the exhaustion, guilt, and sense of endlessness parents face in caring for a technology-dependent child. He described the role confusion they experience as they "breach boundaries of intimacy, inflict pain and confront self-pity and perceptions of futility" (p. 166). Coping abilities worsened over time among the families of eighteen northern California ventilator-dependent children living at home (Quint et al. 1990).

When advanced technology is used in the home to keep alive those who have no reasonable hope of improving, questions of its appropriateness are raised (Belkin 1993; Wolfe et al. 1983). The mother of a 2-year-old with a severe motility disorder ended her child's TPN because she came to feel it was a "means of extraordinary life support" (Strobel et al. 1978).

The burdens of living with technology in the home add to the enormous impact of chronic illness itself on children, parents, siblings, the marriage, and other family systems (Sabbeth 1984). Families accept huge risks taking their technology-dependent children home to live under conditions in which the consequences of human or mechanical failure are potentially fatal (Lantos and Kohrman 1991). The burden of responsibility for these risks shifts from the hospital staff to the family upon discharge home (Lantos and Kohrman 1992). The positive psychological consequences of home care on the child and family, Kohrman (1992) concluded, may be "mitigated or overridden" (p. 164) by these sorts of concerns.

The Costs of High-Tech Home Care for Children

The charges and costs for care at home have consistently been determined to be far less than those for care in the hospital (Bisset et al. 1992; Burr et al. 1983; Pinney and Cotton 1976; Byrne et al. 1979; Feldman and Tuteur 1982; Goldberg et al. 1984; Splaingard et al. 1983), except when the need for nursing care approaches twenty-four hours per day (Aday, Aitken, and Wegener 1988; Frates et al. 1985).

Private insurance fails to cover many expenses related to the care of technology-dependent children. Parents often need to meet high deductibles or make large copayments on expenses that are covered in part. The maximal spending limits of these policies are within easy reach of many of these families. Parents who are able to work remain "wage slaves" to their employers, staying in less desirable jobs simply to retain health insurance premiums for their children's coverage (Freedman and Clarke 1991).

C. Everett Koop was involved as a pediatric surgeon in the development of the home ventilator program in Philadelphia and later, as U.S. Surgeon General, in the passage of the Katie Beckett Waiver and related legislation. In 1982, he convened a two-day workshop, "Children with Handicaps and Their Families," focused on the needs of technology-dependent children. Its goals were to plan a systems approach to health care for ventilator-dependent children, to study the paradigm of dependency on technology, and to develop strategies for organizing and providing care in a cost-effective manner. As a consequence of this workshop, the Division of Maternal and Child Health awarded several grants to encourage the development of regional models of high-tech home care and to evaluate outcomes.

These awards funded an examination of the costs of home ventilator use in children in two studies. In the first, costs in the hospital and at home were compared among thirty-six children from three specialized programs in the United States (Aday, Aitken, and Wegener 1988). To calculate the cost of care in the hospital, the group tallied hospital charges, approximate costs of physician and nursing services, and indirect costs borne by the family. To determine the cost of care at home, it used the actual charges for home-based nursing services, therapies, doctors' visits, equipment rentals, materials, medications, hospital readmissions, administrative costs of home care programs, and some additional costs to parents. After adjustment to reduce possible sources of bias and inaccurate estimation, the group concluded that in 1988 dollars, hospital costs exceeded home care costs by $294 per day ($784 vs. $490 per day). (See chaps. 7 and 13, below for analyses of home care costs for adults on ventilators at home.)

Some cost savings were achieved by the performance of fewer laboratory tests and procedures. The principal source of savings across the three programs was the substitution of parental services for professional nursing in the home. The cost to families of this substitution and of lost opportunities to work or run everyday errands, the "opportunity costs," were not quantified. (Daniels discusses this further in chap. 14, below.) For children requiring nursing services around the clock, costs were comparable in the hospital and at home.

Financial problems were the greatest predictor of family and caregiver "stress." The investigators called for attention to these "mutable aspects [of home care] which health care policy can address" and for careful evaluation of nonpecuniary costs to families of their own, parental substitution of nursing duties (Aday, Aitken, and Wegener 1988). The U.S. Office of Technology Assessment report on technology-dependent children (1987) emphasized the extent to which the demand for nursing hours, the most expensive part of home care, depends heavily on the family's willingness and ability to take responsibility for the child's care.

In another study, the costs to a Medicaid Model Waiver Program of care at home for six ventilator-dependent children in Maryland were compared with reimbursable charges for needed services received had these children been placed in a long-term care facility (Fields et al. 1991). Sixty-nine percent of home care reimbursement was for nursing care. Again, opportunity costs for caregivers were not considered. By this analysis, the mean annual savings were $79,000 per patient ($211 per day), close to the figure derived by Aday's group. The authors concluded that the program was highly cost-effective for the state of Maryland, with the potential for $4 million in annual savings for the full-state, fifty-patient program.

In most states, publicly funded high-tech home care can be initiated for a patient only if it can be projected to cost less than institutional care for that patient. Children requiring extensive nursing services or whose care for any reason is anticipated to cost more at home than in the hospital are therefore unlikely to be discharged to a home care program. This condition is a source of potential selection bias in studies of the comparable costs of home and hospital care, which together with the failure to quantify opportunity costs for caregivers, has led us to underestimate greatly the costs of home care.

Prerequisites to Home Care

Several conditions must be met before a technology-dependent child can be considered ready for discharge from the hospital. The home care plan must be affordable for the family. Funding for medical and nursing care, therapists, equipment, supplies, medication, and transportation must be secured before discharge.

The child must be medically stable (Goldberg, 1992; OTA 1987). No new complications of TPN or ventilator setting changes can be foreseen. The child must be behaviorally manageable, and must not eat the catheter, pull out the tracheostomy tube, or change the dials on the ventilator. The child must be able to swallow medications, accept other treatments, and permit care by people other than the primary caregivers. (Pfister and Pousada discuss discharge planning further in chaps. 4 and 7, below, respectively.)

Equipment must be simple, reliable, and able to be backed up if it fails. It must have adequate alarms, and parents must know how to respond to them. Equipment vendors must provide consistent, dependable service. Home health agencies must be accessible and have experience with technology-dependent children. Skilled nursing caregivers must be available in the home for sufficient numbers of hours. Homemakers and home health aides may need to be employed.

Families must have back-up for the primary caregiver in the event of an emergency. They may need to relocate or renovate their homes to have adequate space and electrical wiring for equipment (Bisset et al. 1992). They should live in clean conditions and in neighborhoods that home-visiting professionals find safe. They must have the ability and desire to understand and accept the risks of taking their child home (O'Leary et al. 1979; OTA 1987; Pinney and Cotton 1976).

There must be adequate transportation to and from medical offices, therapists, and school (OTA 1987). Emergency services must be available to respond in life-threatening situations and transport the child to an appropriate facility. Utility and telephone services must not be cut off immediately in the event of late payment (Sullivan-Bolyai 1991).

The home care of technology-dependent children is ideally coordinated by a multidisciplinary team whose members share their time, skills, and availability (Foster and Hoskins 1981; AAP 1984; Amarnath, Fleming, and Pernault 1987; Goldberg et al. 1984; Goldberg, Gardner, and Gibson 1994; Stein and Jessop 1984a). The team should direct or be closely involved in its patients' acute care and hospital admissions. It can coordinate teaching and training efforts for the family and interpret specialists' opinions and recommendations. It can screen for psychological and social difficulties and either offer appropriate services or refer patients to accessible, capable providers. One such inner-city hospital-based team, the Pediatric Home Care Program, enhanced children's psychological adjustment to chronic illness over the short and long term, compared with standard care in an outpatient clinic (Stein and Jessop 1984b, 1991).

Prescribed pediatric extended care centers offer health care and day programs in the community for children who require sophisticated medical treatment (Pierce, Lester, and Fraze 1991). Developmental planning and parental training are undertaken with a family-centered focus, and highly skilled nursing and therapies (speech, occupational, physical, respiratory) are provided on site. Primary care is coordinated by the center. These types of program should be sought whenever available in the community.

Alternatives to Home Care

Families with technology-dependent children have few alternatives to home or hospital care. The foster care system in the United States is overwhelmed with the needs of children from abusive and neglectful environments. Few foster families have training or expertise in the care of children with chronic conditions. Those who do tend to be asked to care for one or more such children and can rarely take on another. Foster families may need to negotiate different medical, social, and home health care systems for each child with ongoing health needs.

Skilled nursing and intermediate care facilities require that patients be completely stable before admission. Transitional "stepdown" units such as the Polio Respiratory Rehabilitative programs of the 1950s and the units at Children's Hospital of Pennsylvania, Blythedale Children's Hospital in Valhalla, N.Y., and La Rabida Children's Hospital in Chicago require fairly stable children. Their goals are to train caregivers, usually parents, for home care. As extensions of inpatient units, they may provide all or some follow-up medical care or need to arrange for those services upon discharge.

Even when most prerequisites are met, life at home with a technology-dependent child may not work out. Families' needs and supports change over time. The decision to carry out or continue care at home must remain open to renegotiation at all times without an undue burden of shame or guilt on the caregivers (Lantos and Kohrman 1991). Depending on the community, technology-dependent children may be able to enter respite environments on a temporary basis in others' homes, special camps, hospitals, or other institutions. All families must consider these alternatives from time to time (Frates, Harrison, and Splaingard 1984).

Conclusion

High-tech home care supports thousands of children in this country. The survival rates for critically ill children continue to rise. Our inclination to incorporate increasingly sophisticated technology into our everyday lives seems unlikely to turn around soon. Current market forces greatly support the growth of nursing, equipment, and servicing agencies that provide everything required in the home but the parents themselves. For all these reasons, the use of advanced technology in children's homes is likely to expand.

As hospital care improved in the 1970s and 1980s, the inception of many specialized home care programs was prompted by the flood of new survivors of neonatal and pediatric intensive care units and their overwhelming need for care. Program development largely preceded research on the safety and effectiveness of high-tech home care (Lantos and Kohrman 1991). We have not been able to sort out the separate effects on the child and family of chronic illness, hospitalizations, the interventions of home health workers, and having tertiary care equipment in the living room. The impact of high-tech home care seems to be enormous, but we are far from an empiric understanding of the reasons why.

The U.S. Congress Office of Technology Assessment (1987) concluded in its report that there was no concrete evidence for the effectiveness of home care over hospital or institutional care for children dependent on technology. The same can be said of its risks, benefits, and burdens. Biased studies addressing the financial aspects of home care have minimized important elements of its costs. We need to understand all these outcomes, the true costs of this sort of home care, before we expand it further.

To accomplish this, we will need to compare the efficacy, risks, benefits, burdens, and costs of high-tech care in the home with those of care in a variety of institutional settings. We will need to examine social, psychological, and economic outcomes in families who chose either not to use these technologies in the first place or not to take their children home. It is essential that we understand, and not presume we know, the effects of what we do.

REFERENCES

Aday, L. A., Aitken, M. J., and Wegener, D. H. 1988. *Pediatric Home Care: Results of a National Evaluation of Programs for Ventilator Assisted Children.* University of Chicago, Center for Health Administration Studies, Continuing CHAS Research Series, no. 36. Chicago: Pluribus.

Alcock, A. J. W., Hildes, J. A., Kaufert, P. A., Kaufert, J. M., and Bickford, J. 1984. Respiratory poliomyelitis: A follow-up study. *Canadian Medical Association Journal* 130:1305–10.

Alexander, M. A., Johnson, E. W., Petty, J., and Stauch, D. 1979. Mechanical ventilation of patients with late stage Duchenne muscular dystrophy: Management in the home. *Archives of Physical Medicine and Rehabilitation* 60:289–92.

Amarnath, R. P., Fleming, C. R., and Pernault, J. 1987. Home parenteral nutrition in chronic intestinal diseases: Its effect on growth and development. *Journal of Pediatric Gastroenterology and Nutrition* 6:89–95.

American Academy of Pediatrics (AAP) Ad Hoc Task Force on Home Care of Chronically Ill Infants and Children. 1984. Guidelines for Home Care of Infants, Children and Adolescents with Chronic Disease. *Pediatrics* 74:434–36.

Belkin, L. 1993. The High Cost of Living. *New York Times Magazine,* 31 January 1993.

Bisset, W. M., Stapleford, P., Long, S., Chamberlain, A., Sokel, B., and Milia, P. J. 1992. Home parenteral nutrition in chronic intestinal failure. *Archives of Diseases in Childhood* 67:109–14.

Broviac, J. W., Cole, J. J., and Scribner, B. H. 1973. A silicone rubber atrial catheter for prolonged parenteral alimentation. *Surgery, Gynecology and Obstetrics* 136:602.

Broviac, J. W., and Scribner, B. H. 1974. Prolonged parenteral nutrition in the home. *Surgery, Gynecology and Obstetrics* 139:24–28.

Burr, B. H., Guyer, B., Todres, I. D., Abrahams, B., and Chiodo, T. 1983. Home care for children on respirators. *New England Journal of Medicine* 309:1319–23.

Byrne, W. J., Ament, M. E., Burke, M., and Fonkalsrud, E. 1979. Home parenteral nutrition. *Surgery, Gynecology and Obstetrics* 149:593–99.

Byrne, W. J., Halpin, T. C., Asch, M. J., Fonkalsrud, E. W., and Ament, M. E. 1977. Home total parenteral nutrition: An alternative approach to the management of children with severe chronic small bowel disease. *Journal of Pediatric Surgery* 12:359–66.

Cane, R. D., and Shapiro, B. A. 1985. Mechanical ventilatory support. *JAMA* 254:87–92.

Cannon, R. A., Byrne, W. J., Ament, M. E., Gates, B., O'Connor, M., and Fonkalsrud, E. W. 1980. Home parenteral nutrition in infants. *Journal of Pediatrics* 96:1098–1104.

Decker, M. D., and Edwards, K. M. 1988. Central venous catheter infections. *Pediatric Clinics of North America* 35:579–612.

Dorney, S. F. A., Ament, M. E., Berquist, W. E., Vargas, J. H., and Hassall, E. 1985. Improved survival in very short bowel of infancy with use of long-term parenteral nutrition. *Journal of Pediatrics* 107:521–25.

Drinker, P., and Shaw, L. A. 1929. The use of a new apparatus for the prolonged administration of artificial respiration, 1: A fatal case of poliomyelitis. *JAMA* 92:1658–60.

Dudrick, S. J. 1981. A clinical review of nutritional support of the patient. *American Journal of Clinical Nutrition* 34:1191–98.

Dudrick, S. J., Wilmore, D. W., Vars, H. M., and Rhoads, J. E. 1968. Long-term total parenteral nutrition with growth, development and positive nitrogen balance. *Surgery* 64:134–42.

Dudrick, S. J., Wilmore, D. W., Vars, H. M., and Rhoads, J. E. 1969. Can intravenous feeding as the sole means of nutrition support growth in the child and restore weight loss in an adult? An affirmative answer. *Annals of Surgery* 169:974–84.

Dwyer, E., Baker, S. S., and Richardson, D. S. 1987. Home parenteral nutrition. In R. J. Grand, J. L. Sutphen and W. H. Dietz, eds., *Pediatric Nutrition: Theory and practice,* pp. 763–69. Boston: Butterworths.

Engstrom, C. F. 1963. The clinical application of prolonged controlled ventilation. *Acta Anaesthesiol Scand* 8(suppl.):7–52.

Feldman, J., and Tuteur, P. G. 1982. Mechanical ventilation: From hospital intensive care to home. *Heart and Lung* 11:162–165.

Fields, A. I., Rosenblatt, A., Pollack, M. M., and Kaufman, J. 1991. Home care cost effectiveness for respiratory technology-dependent children. *American Journal of Diseases of Children* 145:729–33.

Fleming, C. R., McGill, D. B., and Berkner, S. 1977. Home parenteral nutrition as primary therapy in patients with extensive Crohn's disease of the small bowel and malnutrition. *Gastroenterology* 7:1077–81.

Foster, S., and Hoskins, D. 1981. Home care of the child with a tracheostomy tube. *Pediatric Clinics of North America* 28:855–57.

Frates, R. C., Harrison, G. M., and Splaingard, M. L. 1984. Home care for children on respirators. *New England Journal of Medicine* 310: 1126–27.

Frates, R. C., Splaingard, M. L., Smith, E. O., and Harrison, G. M. 1985. Outcome of home mechanical ventilation in children. *Journal of Pediatrics* 106:850–56.

Freedman, S. A., and Clarke, L. L. 1991. Financing care for medically complex children. In N. J. Hochstadt and D. M. Yost, eds., *The Medically Complex Child: The Transition to Home Care*, pp. 259–86. Chur: Harwood.

Goldberg, A. I. 1983. Home care a better life for ventilator-dependent people. *Chest* 84:365.

Goldberg, A. I. 1992. Pediatric high-technology home care. In M. M. Rothkopf and J. Ashkanazi, eds., *Intensive Homecare*, pp. 199–213. Baltimore: Williams & Wilkins.

Goldberg, A. I., Faure, E. A. M., Vaugh, C. J., Snarski, R., and Seleny, F. L. 1984. Home care for life-supported persons: An approach to program development. *Journal of Pediatrics* 104:785–95.

Goldberg, A. I., Gardner, H. G., and Gibson, L. E. 1994. Home care: The next frontier of pediatric practice. *Journal of Pediatrics* 125:686–90.

Goldberg, A. I., Kettrick, R. G., Buzdygan, D., Lis, E. F., Schraeder, B., and Vaughn, C. 1980. Home ventilation program for infants and children. *Critical Care Medicine* 8:238.

Goldberger, J. H., DeLuca, F. G., Wesselhoeft, C. W., and Randall, H. T. 1979. A home program of long-term total parenteral nutrition in children. *Journal of Pediatrics* 94:325–28.

Goulet, O. J., Revillon, Y, Jan, D., De Potter, S., Maurage, C., Lortat-Jacob, S., Martelli, H., Nihoul-Fekete, C. and Ricour, C. 1991. Neonatal short bowel syndrome. *Journal of Pediatrics* 119:18–23.

Harrison, G. M., and Mitchell, M. B. 1961. The medical and social outcome of 200 respirator and former respirator patients on home care. *Archives of Physical Medicine and Rehabilitation* 4:590–98.

Heird, W. C. 1987. Parenteral nutrition. In R. J. Grand, J. L. Sutphen, and W. H. Dietz, eds., *Pediatric Nutrition: Theory and Practice*, pp. 747–61. Boston: Butterworths.

Helfrick, F. W., and Abelson, N. M. 1944. Intravenous feeding of a complete diet in a child: Report of a case. *Journal of Pediatrics* 25:400–403.

Huddleston, K., Creedmore, P., and Wood, B. 1994. Administration of infant formula through the intravenous route: Consequences and prevention. *American Journal of Maternal/Child Nursing* 19:40–42.

Jeejeebhoy, K. N., Langer, B., Tsallas, G., Chu, R. C., Kuskis, A., and Anderson, G. H. 1976. Total parenteral nutrition at home: Studies in patients surviving four months to five years. *Gastroenterology* 71:943–53.

Kohrman, A. F. 1992. Psychological Issues. In M. J. Mehlman and

S. J. Youngner, eds., *Delivering High Technology Home Care*, pp. 160–78. New York: Springer.

Lantos, J. D., and Kohrman, A. F. 1991. Ethical aspects of pediatric home care. In N. J. Hochstadt and D. M. Yost, eds., *The Medically Complex Child: The Transition to Home Care*, pp. 245–58. Chur: Harwood.

———. 1992. Ethical aspects of pediatric home care. *Pediatrics* 89:920–24.

Lassen, H. C. A. 1953. A preliminary report on the 1952 epidemic poliomyelitis in Copenhagen with special reference to the treatment of acute respiratory insufficiency. *Lancet* 1:37.

Markel, H. 1994. The genesis of the iron lung: Phillip Drinker, Charles F. McKhann, James L. Wilson and early attempts on administering artificial respiration to patients with poliomyelitis. *Archives of Pediatrics and Adolescent Medicine* 148:1174–80.

O'Leary, J., King, R., Leblanc, M., Moss, R., Liebhaber, M., and Lewiston, N. 1979. Cuirass ventilation in childhood neuromuscular disease. *Journal of Pediatrics* 94:419–21.

Palfrey, J. S., Walker, D. K., Haynie, M., Singer, J. D., Porter, S., Bushey, B., and Coopeman, P. 1991. Technology's children: Report of a statewide census of children dependent on medical supports. *Pediatrics* 87:611–18.

Pierce, P. M., Lester, D. G., and Fraze, D. E. 1991. Prescribed pediatric extended care: The family centered health care alternative for medically and technology dependent children. In N. J. Hochstadt and D. M. Yost, eds., *The Medically Complex Child: The Transition to Home Care*, pp. 177–90. Chur: Harwood.

Pinney, M. A., and Cotton, E. K. 1976. Home management of bronchopulmonary dysplasia. *Pediatrics* 58:856–59.

Pitt, H. A., Mann, L. L., Berquist, W. E., Ament, M. E., Fonkalsrud, E. W., and DenBensten, L. 1985. Chronic intestinal psuedo-obstruction: Management with total parenteral nutrition and a venting enterostomy. *Archives of Surgery* 120:614–18.

Pokorny, W. J., Black, C. T., McGill, C. W., Splaingard, M. L., Farrison, G. M., and Harberg, F. J. 1987. Central venous catheters in older children. *Americal Surgeon* 530:524–27.

Quint, R. D, Chesterman, E., Crain, L. S., Winkleby, M., and Boyce, W. T. 1990. Home care for ventilator dependent children: Psychosocial impact on the family. *American Journal of Diseases of Children* 144:1238–41.

Ralston, C. W., O'Connor, M. J., Ament, M., Berquist, W., and Parmelee, A. H. 1984. Somatic growth and developmental functioning in children receiving prolonged home total parenteral nutrition. *Journal of Pediatrics* 105:842–46.

Ricour, C., Gorski, A. M., Goulet, O., de Potter, S., Corriol, O., Postaire, M., Nihoul-Fekete, C., Revillon, Y., Sortat-Jacob, S., and Pellerin, D. 1990. Nutrition in children: Eight years of experience with 112 patients. *Clinical Nutrition* 9:65–71.

Ruben, R. J., Newton, L., Jornsay, D., Stein, R., Chambers, H., Liquori, J., and Lawrence, C. 1982. Home care of the pediatric patients with a tracheostomy. *Annals of Otology, Rhinology and Laryngology* 91:633–40.

Sabbeth, B. 1984. Understanding the impact of chronic childhood illness on families. *Pediatric Clinics of North America* 31:47–58.

Scribner, B. H., Cole, J. J., Christopher, G., Vizzo, J. E., Atkins, R. C., and Blagg, C. R. 1970. Long-term total parenteral nutrition: The concept of an artificial gut. *JAMA* 212:457–63.

Snider, G. I. 1989. Historical perspective on mechanical ventilation: From simple life support system to ethical dilemma. *American Review of Respiratory Diseases* 140:S2-S7.

Splaingard, M. L., Frates, R. C., Harrison, G. M., Carter, R. E., and Jefferson, L. S. 1983. Home positive-pressure ventilation: Twenty years of experience. *Chest* 84:376–82.

Stein, R. E. K., and Jessop, D. J. 1984a. General issues in the care of children with chronic physical illness. *Pediatric Clinics of North America* 31:189–98.

———. 1984b. Does pediatric home care make a difference for children with chronic illness?: Findings from the Pediatric Ambulatory Care Treatment Study. *Pediatrics* 73:845–53.

———. 1991. Long-term mental health effects of a pediatric home care program. *Pediatrics* 88:490–96.

Stern, L., Ramos, A. D., Outerbridge, E. W., and Beaudry, P. H. 1970. Negative pressure artificial respiration: Use in treatment of respiratory failure of the newborn. *Canadian Medical Association Journal* 102:595–601.

Strobel, C. T. 1970. Home parenteral nutrition in children with Crohn's disease. *Gastroenterology* 77:1364.

Strobel, C. T., Byrne, W. J., and Ament, M. E. 1979. Home parenteral nutrition in children with Crohn's disease: An effective management alternative. *Gastroenterology* 77:272–79.

Strobel, C. T., Byrne, W. J., Fonkalsrud, E. W., and Ament, M. E. 1978. Home parenteral nutrition: Results in 34 pediatric patients. *Annals of Surgery* 188:394–402.

Sullivan-Bolyai, S. 1991. The nurse's role: Discharging special needs children to foster care. In N. J. Hochstadt and D. M. Yost, eds., *The Medically Complex Child: The Transition to Home Care*, pp. 81–100. Chur: Harwood.

U.S. Congress, Office of Technology Assessment (OTA). 1987. *Technology-dependent Children: Hospital v. Home Care. A Technical Memorandum.* OTA-5M-H-38. Washington, D.C.: U. S. Government Printing Office.

Vargas, J. H., Ament, M. E., and Berquist, W. E. 1987. Long-term home parenteral nutrition in pediatrics: Ten years of experience in 102 patients. *Journal of Pediatric Gastroenterology and Nutrition* 6:24–32.

Weber, T. R., Tracy, T., and Connors, R.H. 1991. Short bowel syndrome in children: Quality of life in an era of improved survival. *Archives of Surgery* 126:841–46.

Wolfe, B. M., Beer, W. H., Hayashi, J. T., Halsted, C. H., Cannon, R. A., and Cox, K. L. 1983. Experience with home parenteral nutrition. *American Journal of Surgery* 146:7–12.

3. Chimeras and Odysseys

TOWARD UNDERSTANDING THE TECHNOLOGICALLY
DEPENDENT CHILD

Arthur F. Kohrman, M.D.

> Dire chimera's conquest was enjoined;
> the mingled monster, of no mortal kind;
> Behind a dragon's fiery tail was spread;
> A goat's rough body bore a lion's head;
> Her pitchy nostrils flaky flames expire;
> Her gaping throat emits infernal fire.
>
> *The Odyssey*, trans. Alexander Pope

Preserving the lives of children and adults by attaching them for long periods of time to technological devices extends not only the lives of human beings but also the definition of the nature of being human to include human-and-machine combinations. Yet we as individuals, as professionals, and as a society are unclear about the nature or value of these combinations. I see this uncertainty as a potentially fruitful point of departure for this book on the ethical and social implications of high-tech home care. Seeking as we all do to bridge the gap between what we see and what we must but don't know, I found myself turning for help to metaphor. The resort to metaphor in describing technology-dependent children and their families is natural and necessary, because it is most often by metaphor—by common culturally held images and stories—that we collectively understand the new and perplexing, especially when it forces new visions of things so important and universal as children and life itself (Lakoff and Johnson 1981).

Children connected to ventilators evoke the image of chimeric creatures: they are a combination of two different species. I contend that this combination of two historically unrelated conceptual domains—the human and the mechanical—perplexes us and confuses our senses of the identity and value of these human-machine hybrids.

In Bulfinch's *Mythology* (1898), the Chimera is described in the chapter on monsters. In mythology, monsters were (are) beings of unnatural proportions or parts, usually regarded with terror, possessing immense strength and ferocity, which they employed for the injury and annoyance of mortals. Some of them (e.g., the Sphinx and the Chimera) were combinations of parts of different animals; to these were attributed all the terrible qualities of wild beasts as well as human sagacity and feeling, and, in the case of the Sphinx, godlike qualities as well.

Some of the definitions of a chimera in the *Oxford English Dictionary* show the multiplicity of ways we can describe our confusion:

1. A chimera is a fabled fire-breathing monster with a lion's head, a goat's body, and a serpent's tail.
2. A grotesque monster formed with the parts of various animals.
3. With reference to the terrible character, unreal or incongruous composition of the fabled monster: a horrible and fear-inspiring phantasm, an unreal creation of the imagination, a mere wild fantasy, an unfounded conception; an incongruous union.

The Chimera of mythology was a fearful monster breathing fire, with the head of a lion, the body of a goat, and the tail of a dragon. Now visualize for a moment a child: a quadriplegic, ventilator-dependent child . . . head of a lion, the (partially or completely useless) body of a goat, and—the tail of a dragon—the real technological tether, the tubes connecting the child to the ventilator and its alarm devices. ("Her pitchy nostrils flaky flames expire; Her gaping throat emits infernal fire.")

Anyone who has tried to replace a tracheotomy tube in a struggling child who is totally dependent on a ventilator can identify all the elements. It is truly terrifying to see the child struggle as the seconds of breathlessness pass while the caregiver desperately but meticulously tries to insert a tracheotomy tube into a secretion-filled trachea—the "gaping throat amidst the infernal fire."

The Chimera of mythology made havoc in the kingdom, so the king, Iobates, sought a hero to destroy it. That hero was Bellerophon, who, by a series of events, ended up in the court of Iobates, carrying with him a decree the last line of which was that Iobates should kill him. Iobates gave Bellerophon a series of tests, hoping that he would fail and must then be put to death. One of the tests was to kill the Chimera. Bellerophon went to sleep in the temple of Minerva, and, in a dream, Minerva brought to him a golden bridle, which he used the next day to mount the winged horse Pegasus; he then flew off and easily conquered the Chimera. Bellerophon passed test after test until "at length, Iobates, seeing that the hero was a special favorite of the gods, gave him his daughter in marriage and made him his successor on the throne."

This story has, however, an unhappy and perhaps cautionary conclusion: "At last, Bellerophon, by his pride and presumption, drew upon himself the anger of the gods; it is said he even attempted to fly up into heaven on his winged steed; but Jupiter sent a gadfly which stung Pegasus and made him throw his rider, who became lame and blind in consequence" (Bulfinch 1898, p. 157). Thus, Bellerophon, the rescuer (perhaps the physician?) is himself done in by his own arrogance and hubris. Does this metaphor also carry with it the warning to us, the enthusiastic employers and advocates of our technologies, that immoderation leads to unfulfillable expectations and our own downfall?

My basic thesis is that we have no clear image of who or what technology-dependent children are or of who we are as professionals caring for them. Like the Chimera, the new beings, humans attached to and dependent on machines, have created disarray in our ways of thinking; and like Iobates, we are seeking a decisive and heroic way to contain that confusion. We, both professionals and public, seek to recognize and categorize the novel and unfamiliar; indeed, the very art of medical diagnosis is the recognition of groups of similar or related findings. I think we don't really know yet what technology-dependent people are, what known or related prior experiences they best match, or what group to put them into. We seek conceptualizations and meanings of a novel category of persons.

In responding to requests to talk or write about the ethical issues raised by technology-dependent people, I have come to realize that we can't construct an ethical system for something or someone for which or whom we don't understand the meaning or value, and in our society we don't yet know how we value technology-dependent people. Until we have a clearer idea of what they are and what they mean to us collectively and as professionals, we will be unable to answer clearly even the basic operational questions that arise in and from their care and presence. I have not yet found a common or cohesive understanding of what a technology-dependent child is. Is it a child connected to a machine, with all the endearing, dependent, hopeful characteristics of childhood? For most of us who, after all, are engaged in humanistic pursuits, this is the most necessary and compelling view. But that view is constantly strained by the necessity to tend to the machines, lest the child perish. Thus we often find ourselves behaving as if the beast is a machine supporting a child. If the machine and its performance are the critical focus of concern, a device originally used as a means becomes an end in itself.

Is the child-machine combination a being in its own right, or just a stage of a medically engineered metamorphosis—a cocoon from which we wait hopefully for the real, intact child to emerge? Or is it an arrested metamorphosis, from which the child can go neither forward nor backward, but commands endless attention in some sort of ensnaring connection with those who must watch and care for it? At various times and phases in the journey of each child toward independence from the technology, if it is to be achieved, the technology-dependent child is all of these. Each of the conceptualizations has unique challenges and fears and demands unique responses, evolving with the changing condition of the child.

Some of the most important tasks of development in children are those of distinguishing self from others and achieving independence. How do we (and the child) understand the boundaries of self in a child who is connected to a machine? And how do we mark and define maturation and development in a child dependent for survival itself on that machine, when the common benchmarks for those qualities have to do with increasing independence and autonomy? What are the anthropomorphic concepts of the machine held by these children and by those who help them? Think about the popular toys called "transformers," toys that a child can turn from machines into human figures and back again. I wonder how children connected to a machine see themselves in that transformation.

How do these children understand their relationship to the technology? Do they see the machines as part of their bodies? Does the machine overpower the child, or alternatively, might it give the child a greater sense of worth or singularity: "Hey, look at me!" One of the children known to us uses his connection to a ventilator as an opening line in a stand-up comic act. Clearly, for each child the answers to these questions will be unique, as the developmental pathway and the unfolding sense of self is unique for all children; yet we are puzzled about the reasonable expectations for development, discipline, and progress.

And what of those whose lives, by choice or circumstance, are tethered to the child-machine creature? Are they servants, slaves, angels—are they blessed or cursed? One of the accomplishments of successful parenting is the facilitation of the separation of the child, but for these children separation may mean death.

How do parents mirror their child's own sense of bodily integration? We all become very concerned when one of our children is hurt or ill, and we work to reestablish both for the child and for ourselves the sense of the child's wholeness after the illness or injury is over. How do parents find that wholeness and recovery when their child is permanently hooked up to a machine, a machine whose failure or malfunction can bring injury or death to the child? Many acts of everyday life, like being held, are so important to a child. What is it like to hold a child on a ventilator, listening to the damnable thing wheezing twenty-four hours a day, with the endless rattle of secretions in the child's tracheotomy? Such an experience is hardly part of the anticipations of child-rearing.

How will a society so dependent on machinery view these children? Where would we be without our beepers, our fax machines, our telephones? Yet we don't ordinarily consider these to be extensions of our bodies, even though we often joke about how we could not live without them or we can't imagine how we lived before them. If we look analytically at how we use them, they are, in fact, extensions of our working bodies, but we know that our dependence on them is chosen. No such choice exists for the individual for whom technology is truly life-sustaining. In any real sense of threat to existence itself, it is false (and trivializing) to talk in the same breath about our optional everyday mechanical dependences and the obligate dependence of children on ventilators or other life-preserving devices, yet how must those jokes and conversations feel to them and their caregivers? Where do these two kinds of dependence on technology blend, and where do they diverge in the minds of the child, the parents, and the professionals? How do the parents of technology-dependent children see the question of service maintenance? There is a certain kind of dark, latent humor in the idea of a "40,000-breath check-up." For whom is it done, the child or the machine? Do they go to the shop together?

These are the kinds of question we must ask if we are going to really talk about and with technology-dependent children and adults, and their caregivers and families, as human beings. The answers to some of these questions lie in further research on the now-considerable numbers of children and their families who have experienced technology dependence and assistance over several years; the answers to others will need to be found anew for each child and family as they face their particular realities and futures.

Why must we grapple with these descriptive questions? Because we cannot make rational individual or collective social judgments about what we cannot describe, and we cannot construct a moral and political framework for something whose value and meaning we don't know. Children who are technology dependent and their caregivers are torn between competing and confusing forces and constructs. The challenges to successful development of an intact child are formidable enough; the conflicts, uncertainties, and tensions between dependence and growing independence are daunting. In addition to the uncertainties of effective child-rearing, parents of technology-dependent children are caught in the web of conflicts between their commitment and moral reason and the realities of the political and social worlds they live in. The differences between what is and what ought to be are a life theme for these children and families.

Unquestionably, those who care for others whose lives depend on technology have a fundamental desire to succeed in that difficult task, and their actions are driven by the most fundamental principles of love, the maintenance of life for vulnerable humans, and the exercise of exemplary professional competence. However, while firm in their own commitments to the individuals in their care, they face a society that may not share their commitment and their uncertainty about the best and most humane ways to pursue their tasks. Ultimately, their decisions and choices, as those of the larger society, will be determined by their fundamental values; that is, how they see what is best and desirable for themselves and their charges. Their decisions, in turn, will inevitably be conditioned by the available resources and support, emotional and tangible, in their immediate surroundings and in the social and political environment.

Thus, in our journey toward an ethical framework for the consideration of technology-dependent persons we arrive first at an analysis of values. In this exercise, I would like to examine the definitions of *value*, which I believe are confused in the discussion about technology-dependent children. In our everyday language we conflate two distinctive uses of the word *value*. The first is the use of values to define a hierarchy of preferences or choices, which guide social decision-making and political behavior. The second definition of *value* is what something is worth or what it costs (not always the same!). We tend to use these definitions somewhat loosely; for this discussion of children dependent on technology, we must be more precise, because each of the definitions has important conceptual and rhetorical consequences as we attempt to understand the relatively new chimeric species.

For the moment I wish to speak about values as the choices and preferences, social and political, that determine how people act as individuals or collectively, as a society. Using that definition, I assert that our culture is not particularly hospitable to (a) children; (b) children with chronic illness; or (c) particularly, children who are technology dependent. What are the most prized values—if you will, virtues—in our culture that are inimical to technology-dependent children? They include individualism, physical beauty (and the narcissism that goes with it), physical and social mobility, the ability to compete, and independence. Of these, independence is the one most clearly affronted by the technology-dependent person, but each of them is in some degree compromised in the lives of all disabled people, and especially those who are technology dependent. Thus, we are talking about those who, by definition, are likely to be devalued in their own society.

Then, another set of values is held by the professionals and embedded throughout the culture of medicine. Medical professionals reflect in their behaviors their preference for cure, for brief encounters with clear outcomes, and for evident, progressive improvement by the patient. We professionals reward self-help and tend to think less of those who do not appear to be struggling to get better, even when the circumstances of their disability or illness prohibit such a struggle: we believe that those who really want to get better will (and can) work in their own behalf to do so. The unwritten text is that if sick or disabled people don't get better, it is because they didn't try hard enough. Technology-dependent persons come up against all of those professional values (many of which are also embedded in the larger cultural view of medicine) in addition to the often hostile values of the larger society itself.

If we turn, then, to the challenges to technology-dependent children, we see them falling short of the desirable at many levels. They rarely, or only very slowly, get better; they often can't help themselves; they are not fully independent and may never be so; they often are not "beautiful" in the usual sense (indeed, they are sometimes fearsome to look at). They present an unfamiliar image and presence that can evoke very deep concerns, even fear or revulsion. Such negative reactions to these individuals and the emotions they invoke may be very powerful but not acknowledged by the public, by the child's caregivers, by the children themselves, or by the involved professionals.

Technology-dependent individuals challenge many of the values of the society and of the professional establishments. This reality places these children and their caregivers in a very vulnerable position in an environment where choices are made by political processes that ultimately reflect the dominant social values. There is a real risk that those political choices that determine the allocation of restricted resources will disfavor those for whom technology is critical, unless those of us who are committed to them remain vigilant and active in the political arenas where decisions about resource allocation are made.

A second common meaning of *value* is that of cost. Technology-dependent children and adults are expensive individuals in our society. They are not more expensive than weapons or cosmetics or some of the other things we as a country and individuals spend large sums of money on, but they are expensive in the range of ordinary medical and social endeavors. One of the issues that rattles about in the political arena is the aggregate cost of caring for these individuals over time. Compared with that of other populations at risk (e.g., elderly people), the aggregate cost is not great because their numbers are not great. But they stand out egregiously in individual case-expense calculations, and the costs of their care are often used to create a political sense of their "burden" to society that far outweighs its real economic weight.

Another kind of worth, clearly more important, must also be acknowledged: moral worth. What it is worth to our society to keep such individuals alive and optimally supported? Technology-dependent persons bring us face to face with the very basic issue of who are deserving and who are undeserving. What do these people and their care mean for our collective understanding of the nature of being human; what moral cost would there be in abandoning their support and care? One of the embedded tenets of American society is our inclination to measure our society's integrity by how we take care of those who are least well off—a kind of irreducible bottom line of social responsibility. If we begin explicitly negotiating that floor by determining *de jure* that some of the least well off are not worthy of our efforts, have we done irreparable harm?

Finally, the definition of *value* as tangible worth becomes a useless and bedeviling descriptor for this population. How much is a $3000 respirator worth when it is hooked up to a child? Money becomes meaningless in any real moral or even operational sense, but discussions of money dominate political decision-making. Those of us who work with and advocate for those whose lives depend on technology must constantly counter those political assertions that divert the discussion from the more thorny issues of moral worth to the simplistic and meaningless (even destructive) ones of tangible worth.

Moreover, since we can't quantify in tangible terms the worth of these individuals, we may instead ask whether they are important to us as icons, as symbols. As a nation, we have made a massive commitment to elderly people in the form of Medicare. We have no comparable commitment to children. Are technology-dependent children the most dependent, the most compelling symbols for the plight of all children in our society? Elderly people are not simply icons, and I suspect that these children are not just icons either. They have many complicated moral connections to our society and its values across *all* the definitions of *value* I have explored.

There is much to be learned about these people whose destiny and even survival are tied to machines: about how they see themselves, how they see a perplexed and possibly hostile world, and how that world sees, values, and, ultimately, treats them. It will take many years, even generations, before their presence is accepted as just another variation of human form and identity. We can only speculate about their futures in a world where, on one hand, there is increasing acceptance of persons with disabilities as full citizens and, on the other, tribalism and the hatred of those unlike the dominant groups is the justification for mass exclusion and even murder. One can guess that, as with other new human endeavors, the future for technology-dependent people will be mixed and that acceptance and accommodation will coexist with continued exclusion and denials of their essential humanity.

We cannot abandon, however, our efforts to know better what these people mean—for us, for themselves, for society—as if their situations had no parallels in our collective experience from which we might draw guidance or, at least, reassurance. That collective experience is not only the history of world and human events but also the record of human foolishness and triumph in the face of the unexpected and previously unknown. Much of the history of all cultures and their views and values is embedded and transmitted in stories and myths, the metaphorical repositories of wisdom and experience, and it is often through and in those old metaphors that we can find some ways to begin thinking about the new and unfamiliar.

Technical descriptions of devices and their use, the recitations of the joys and burdens of caring for technology-dependent people, or even being one of them, are by themselves insufficient to bring us, as individuals and as a society, to a realization of the meaning of this truly new creature made up of humans and machines intertwined and interdependent in so many ways. If the person-machine combination can be understood in part as a modern-day chimera, and some of our reactions to it revealed through our reading of mythology, it may be similarly useful to look into other allegories and metaphors. Is the child supported by a ventilator not really also like another of the mythical creatures, the Sphinx, offspring of Chimera, with its woman's head, bird's wings and claws, and lion's body? The riddle of the Sphinx—what animal has four feet in the morning, two at noon, and three at night?—is a riddle for the child's caregivers as well. Oedipus succeeded in overcoming the Sphinx by solving the riddle, recognizing that each stage represented a step in the progress of humans through life: four-legged at infancy, two-legged in adulthood, three-legged (with a cane) in old age. Children dependent on technologies similarly present to their parents an enigma, a riddle that must be solved so that both can exist. And like the riddle of the Sphinx, the answer and the triumph lie in understanding development and growth in unfamiliar terms.

Another figure in mythology made up of parts of two species is the centaur. Unlike other such creatures, the centaur held favored status among both gods and humans. One centaur in particular, the wise and learned Chiron, stands out. Chiron, known for his great healing powers and knowledge of medicine, educated both Hercules and Jason. Thus, this gentle man-beast both introduced his pupils to knowledge and launched each of them on daring, challenging, extraordinary, and heroic life-defining journeys—Hercules to his daunting and exceptional tasks, and Jason to his pursuit of the Golden Fleece. How much this is like the child-machine, challenging parents and caregivers to unimagined tasks and journeys and rewards, and, in the process, elevating them to the ranks of heroes!

The journey of the parents of a technology-dependent child is truly an Odyssey, and their experiences are nowhere better understood than through the trials of Odysseus, beginning with his encounter with Circe, the enchantress who changes humans into beasts, a metaphor for the transformation of a child into a potentially frightening new species of being. The entrapment of Odysseus in Cyclops's cave reminds us of the endlessness and terror in caring for a child dependent on not only machines but also on the vigilance of those who watch the machines. Parents must face and deal with the prognostications of physicians who are guessing at futures for children unlike others they have seen, worrying about and foretelling dire fates for these children at the hands of those who are committed to the preservation of their lives. These ominous prophesies are like those of Tiresias to Odysseus, in which he warned of all the trials and dangers ahead. The cries of the Sirens, so compelling yet so threatening, are to parents and caregivers like the cries of the children asking for relief from the constant mechanical and human presence to which they are bound—sweet and reasonable, and utterly fatal.

The insoluble and endless choices between life for the child and the often grotesque, always intrusive procedures necessary to maintain that life are a constant and endlessly repeated running of the perilous passage between Scylla, the dragon who threatened to destroy Odysseus and his companions, and Charybdis, the whirlpool. The conversion of living rooms and bedrooms into intensive care units is for patients and parents like the experience of Odysseus returning to a home no longer the home remembered; and while the many nurses, technicians, and volunteers technology-dependent children and their parents find in that home cannot be slain or expelled, they need to be subjugated so that a familiar life can be regained, much as Odysseus had to recapture his own home from strangers upon his return.

A recurrent and pervasive strain in all mythology, and especially in the Odyssey, is the interpretation of powerful events and forces as the counterpoint of love and war. Caring for a person who is technology dependent is a modern enactment of these same themes. The love of a parent or companion is constantly tested in the many battles of the home care experience, and sometimes, even with the greatest love, individual battles, and even the war, are lost.

However, like Odysseus, while the journey may seem endless and the challenges daunting, both child and parents can take on heroic stature from just surviving from task to task, from day to day, from challenge to challenge. Will that promise, and the continued or prolonged existence of a person heretofore doomed, be reward enough for the struggle? Unlike the Odyssey, the ending of this contemporary exploration is not yet written, and the judgment of history not within our knowing. This is a brave new world of challenge to those whose lives are bound to technology, their families and caregivers and companions, and those who launch them on their journeys. Will this new world produce new mythical figures for future generations to study and revere? Or will we be judged like Bellerophon, brought to earth by our hubris, to be mocked for attempting to transcend both our humanity and its inevitable end? The context is new, the questions very old.

ACKNOWLEDGMENTS

I wish to thank Linda Diamond Shapiro, who first suggested the chimera analogy; Beth Plunkett, who plumbed mythological sources; and Claire Kohrman, who helped me understand what I wanted to say.

REFERENCES

Bulfinch, T. 1898. *The Age of Fable or Beauties of Mythology*. Philadelphia: David McKay.

Guerber, H. A. 1933. *The Myths of Greece and Rome*. New York: Dover Publications.

Lakoff, G., and Johnson, M. 1981. *Metaphors We Live By*. Chicago: University of Chicago Press.

Oxford English Dictionary. Oxford: Oxford University Press.

4. Oncology and High-Tech Home Care

David G. Pfister, M.D.

When carcinoma in situ and nonmelanoma skin cancers are excluded, approximately 1,100,000 new cases of cancer are diagnosed in the United States each year. Malignant disease accounts for slightly over 500,000 deaths annually, second only to cardiovascular disease (Boring, Squires, and Tong 1991). Despite important advances in certain areas, cancer remains a major source of morbidity and mortality in this country, and cancer patients are major consumers of high-tech and other home care services.

Although the above figures include a broad and heterogeneous spectrum of cancer diagnoses, certain generalizations can be made that help to explain further why cancer is such an important public health concern and a significant influence on the rapidly evolving high-tech home care industry.

1. Many tumors are diagnosed at an advanced stage, and distant metastases are common. These tumors are typically not cured by local therapies such as surgery or radiation. While patients with certain advanced and/or metastatic tumors (e.g., adult and childhood leukemia, lymphoma, childhood sarcoma, testicular cancer) are now routinely cured with the addition of available systemic therapies (Devita 1990), these diseases unfortunately represent less than 10 percent of cancer diagnosed in the United States each year. Solid tumors at four primary sites (lung, colon/rectum, breast, and prostate) account for over 50 percent of the incidence and mortality of cancer in this country (Boring, Squires, and Tong 1991). Available systemic therapies for these latter diseases are typically palliative, not curative.

2. The cancers that are potentially curable by systemic therapy in their advanced stages tend to occur in younger patients. Most other malignancies generally occur in older individuals, with approximately 55 percent of cancer diagnosed in the 13 percent of the U.S. population that is 65 years of age or older (Kennedy 1992). For these older cancer

65 Endicott College

Beverly, Mass. 01915

patients, improvements in survival have been modest at best over the last two to three decades. Not surprisingly then, the concerns of the geriatric and oncologic health care communities often overlap (see chap. 7, below).

3. Many therapies for solid tumors in adults, while not curative, can afford effective palliation for significant periods of time. For example, patients with metastatic prostate or breast cancer have median survivals of two to three years (Clark et al. 1986; Crawford et al. 1989). These patients, when responding to treatment, are much like any other patient with a chronic disease.

4. Many solid tumors in adults are associated with tobacco, alcohol, or other substance abuse (Tuyns 1982; Wynder and Hoffmann 1982). The management of these patients is further complicated by the comorbid ailments associated with these habits and lifestyles.

5. Both conventional and investigational therapeutic modalities available for the treatment of cancer can be associated with a variety of substantial side effects. Although the initial management of these toxicities is often done in the hospital, once stabilized, many patients can have their treatment completed or maintained at home.

Given these general themes, it is not surprising that high-tech home care has many potential areas of application for patients with neoplastic disease. Being at home would presumably facilitate a better quality of life for most of these patients. The development and evolution of the home hospice movement in this country would further confirm this impression. As Schachter and Holland observe in chapter 6 of this volume, many patients, if properly supported, prefer to die at home (Groth-Juncker and McCusker 1983). With patients who are often chronically ill, the exposure to infectious disease that is a risk of any hospitalization can be minimized (Pizzo et al. 1993). Therapies can be delivered less expensively, since the fixed costs associated with delivering care in a hospital are avoided, at least in part. Those patients who are more stable and better candidates for obtaining various services at home generally receive the least attention when hospitalized, since more ill patients dominate the time of the hospital professional staff. Even the most dedicated and compassionate hospital staff cannot provide the type of love, attention, and support potentially provided by devoted family and friends. Finally, from an entrepreneurial perspective, the treatment of the cancer patient represents an important area of potential profit for the high-tech home care industry.

At its inception, high-tech home care mainly focused on intravenous access/hydration and the delivery of parenteral nutrition. Over the last decade, the services have expanded in concert with growing demand and acknowledgment of the feasibility of the approach. The provision of home antibiotics and total parenteral nutrition are the primary anchors of the industry (personal communication, Biomedical Business International, 1992), but many other technologies and services are available. For purposes of this chapter, I focus on certain areas where high-tech home care is commonly used in the oncology population, including intravenous access and the use of portable infusion pumps; pain control; the provision of hydration and nutrition; drug infusion, most commonly for infection (including bone marrow transplant patients) or cancer treatment; and respiratory care. Issues relevant to their application to cancer patients are stressed. Certain technologies are discussed by Okun and Pousada in chapters 2 and 7 of this volume, respectively, and are not reviewed here (e.g., the use of high-tech beds) or are discussed in less detail (e.g., respiratory care).

Specific Topics

As with other diseases, successful use of these technologies in the home with cancer patients involves certain prerequisites. The patient should be in a stable clinical condition. A supportive and involved family or surrogate is important. Both the patient and the other involved individuals must be able to learn the tasks necessary to monitor and use the technology properly. Finally, the patient must have the appropriate insurance and/or financial resources to pay for the expenses of such therapies. This is obviously an important issue, since many patients and their families become financially depleted, if not bankrupt, because of the ongoing and substantial expenses incurred during a long illness.

Intravenous Access/Infusions

The provision of ongoing, easily maintained intravenous access is the common denominator for the provision of many therapies in the home. This is a real challenge in cancer patients, since during the course of their disease, intravenous access typically becomes a progressive problem. Frequent drawing of blood samples, frequent insertion of standard intravenous catheters to facilitate the provision of supportive care and treatment, often for prolonged periods, and the use of vesicant (e.g., anthracyclines, vinca alkaloids) and other locally irritating drugs are all contributory. Traditional intravenous catheters require frequent changing, can clot off or otherwise become nonfunctional at unpredictable times, and become progressively difficult and at times impossible to insert. As patients become more debilitated and symptomatic, the monitoring of blood tests and the use of intravenous therapies will often escalate, further exacerbating the problem. For patients already suffering the physical, psychological, and emotional consequences of the symptoms associated with their underlying malignancy, the discomfort associated with unsuccessful attempts at phlebotomy and the insertion of an intravenous catheter is especially frustrating and burdensome. Important home therapies will often need to be interrupted if easily maintained intravenous access is not available.

The establishment of central venous access is generally used to overcome this problem (Groeger, Lucas, and Coit 1991). Central veins are larger and have increased blood flow, thus minimizing the local irritant effect associated with the various infusions that the patient receives. Patients with short-term requirements are generally managed with the percutaneous placement of a single or multilumen central venous catheter. The drawbacks of these catheters for more chronic use are that sutures or local dressings are the only safeguards to prevent dislodgment, and the vascular-cutaneous tunnel is short, thus increasing the theoretical risk of septicemia. Another option is a peripherally inserted central catheter, or so-called PICC line. This is inserted through the antecubital vein and advanced to a central venous location. Such a line can be placed by a specially trained nurse and be left in place for a long period of time. Obviously, an adequate antecubital venous system is necessary for the insertion of a PICC line.

Two types of surgically inserted silastic catheter, however, are most commonly used when chronic central venous access is needed. Both have been well described elsewhere (Groeger, Lucas, and Coit 1991). The first involves the insertion of a catheter into the subclavian vein, with the distal or external end of the catheter then tunneled through the pectoralis major muscle so that the end used for infusion is both external and distant from the vein-insertion site. This location is also more convenient and comfortable for maintenance and appearance than an exit site higher in the neck. Examples of this type of catheter are the Hickman/Broviac and Groshong catheters. The second type involves the placement of a catheter with a distal end containing a metal septum covered by a membrane that is implanted beneath the skin. The catheter is accessed by inserting a needle through the skin and membrane into the septum. An example of this latter type is the Mediport.

Once placed, both types of catheter can remain in place for

months to years. Maintenance includes local care and periodic flushing with anticoagulant to prevent clotting. The external type is favored for patients who access the port on a frequent basis (e.g., patients with leukemia), since multiple separate ports are commonly needed and repeated skin punctures are not necessary to access the device. The Mediport is otherwise used, as it is under the skin, cosmetically preferable, and easier to maintain. Both types of catheter require implantation by a surgeon. The procedure is relatively minor, and complications (e.g., pneumothorax, infection, bleeding) are infrequent but can be serious. Over time, the catheter can clot off or become a nidus of infection, especially with patients undergoing myelosuppressive chemotherapy, and removal or replacement is necessary. Infection is the culprit in 6 to 27 percent of these cases (Groeger, Lucas, and Coit, 1991). Because of these concerns, other materials that will facilitate longer duration of insertion and less local trauma to peripheral veins are in development.

Another type of technology commonly used in cancer patients that goes hand in hand with the issue of vascular access involves pumps that facilitate the administration of a variety of intravenous therapies in the home. Most commonly used are external pumps. Various types are available, many of which are so portable that patients can be fully ambulatory with them. Depending on the purpose, examples of portable pumps include the Travenol infuser, Pharmacia pump, Cormed pump, and the Autosyringe. Each type varies in the difficulty of operation, cost, and available options. These pumps have been described in more detail and are illustrated elsewhere (Bruera et al. 1987).

Pain Control

Pain is one of the most common complaints in cancer patients, occurring in more than 70 percent of patients with advanced disease (Portenoy 1989). Narcotic analgesics are commonly required to obtain adequate pain control (Cherny and Portenoy 1993). Although oral administration is the preferred route initially, many patients will require parenteral opioids to control their symptoms. These are most commonly administered subcutaneously or intravenously. Cancer pain is frequently chronic, and unfortunately is often undertreated. Concerns regarding the possibility of a narcotic overdose, poor intravenous access and the potential complications associated with a long-term intravenous catheter, the need for frequent nursing assessments, and expensive/complicated infusion pumps are all in part responsible for this syndrome of undertreatment. Prolonged hospitalizations can occur in the absence of the availability of appropriate pain-control technology in the home. A well-orchestrated home care program can effectively deal with these concerns (Coyle et al. 1985). Since many of these patients have incurable disease, prolonged hospitalizations can have an adverse effect on the quality of their remaining time.

Hydration and Nutrition

Weight loss and signs of malnutrition are among the most common findings reported in cancer patients. Depending on the primary site, significant weight loss at presentation is found in 31 to 87 percent of advanced cancer patients participating in chemotherapy trials (De-Wys et al. 1980). Dehydration or malnutrition can arise from a variety of causes in these patients. The appropriate management is dictated by the cause. The problem can be temporary (e.g., treatment-related toxicity, nausea/vomiting) or permanent (short bowel syndrome); it can reflect a local mechanical problem with (e.g., advanced head and neck cancer) or without (e.g., small bowel obstruction from disease and management of ovarian cancer) a functioning gastrointestinal tract. As a general rule, the existing digestive tract is used for nutritional supplementation whenever possible, because of cost and toxicity concerns (Shike 1992).

Simple dehydration of short duration is generally treated with intravenous fluids with salt, other electrolytes, and dextrose. These fluids do not provide complete nutrition, but this is generally not a problem if the poor oral intake resolves promptly. For more sustained problems with oral intake and nutrition in patients with a functioning gastrointestinal tract, a large number and variety of enteral formulas are available that provide balanced nutrition and can be taken by mouth. These formulas (e.g., Ensure, Isocal) can be used to supplement an incomplete diet or as complete nutrition by themselves. Partly digested formulas are available for patients with specific digestion defects. When such formulas cannot be taken in adequate volume by mouth because of local mechanical problems, options to bypass the usual swallowing mechanism are available. The simplest option is the placement of a flexible tube through the nose and into the stomach. The customary nasogastric tube made of polyvinyl chloride is poorly suited for long-term feeding and is uncomfortable for the patient. Nasogastric tubes specifically designed for feeding purposes and longer duration of placement have a narrower caliber, are generally made of polyurethane, have a weighted end, and can be easily advanced into the small intestine. Although easy to place, such feeding tubes can be easily dislodged and are cosmetically least appealing to the patient. An increasingly used alternative, especially for patients with a chronic need for enteral feeding, is the placement of a tube directly into the stomach (gastrostomy) or jejunum (jejunostomy). Historically, an open surgical procedure was necessary to place these tubes. In recent years, a percutaneous endoscopic approach is used in most patients. These tubes can be placed in an outpatient procedure, generally with no or minor complications, and can be easily hidden under usual clothing (Shike et al. 1989). Bolus feedings are used when the tube is placed in the stomach. Infusion feedings requiring a pump are necessary when the tube is in the jejunum or if the patient has a digestive defect requiring slow delivery of formula.

The alternative to an enteral approach is total parenteral nutrition (TPN), whereby all essential nutrition is administered intravenously. TPN is used only in very selected circumstances in which the gastrointestinal tract is not functioning. Examples include patients with short bowel syndrome after an extended resection; patients recovering from radiation enteritis; and patients having problems with bowel obstruction. For long-term administration, central access is required. TPN is more expensive ($299 to $530 dollars per day for two liters of solution, from my own survey of four providers), requires more careful monitoring, and has a greater likelihood of severe complications.

The anorexia associated with systemic carcinomatosis is well described. The administration of TPN to patients with such advanced or end-stage disease is not encouraged. Substantial toxicity is more likely to occur in these debilitated patients, and there is no evidence to suggest that parenteral nutrition significantly improves the quality of life or survival of these patients with such a poor prognosis. The use of oral megestrol acetate may improve the patient's appetite and induce weight gain (Aisner et al. 1990).

Drug Administration: Antibiotics and Chemotherapy

The most common reason for the institution of parenteral antibiotics in the cancer patient is fever with neutropenia (an abnormal drop in the number of white blood cells), often complicated by other documented infection(s) (Pizzo et al. 1993). Although many of these occurrences are uncomplicated, there is always the risk of an evolving, life-threatening infection. At least initially, these patients are generally treated in the hospital, though the possibility of outpatient treatment for selected patients at low risk for developing serious infection is being actively investigated (Rubenstein et al. 1993). If no infection is documented, antibiotics are discontinued when blood counts recover, and the duration of treatment is generally short. Patients are discharged from the hospital without the need for antibiotics, thus additional therapy at home is unnecessary. If an infection is found, generally the treatment lasts no longer than two weeks. While some of these patients when stable complete their antibiotic course at home, many will stay in the hospital for the duration of their therapy. Antimicrobial therapy at home is particularly well suited for situations in which the patient is stable after initial treatment, and longer durations of treatment (four to six weeks) are necessary, such as in the therapy of bone (osteomyelitis) or heart valve (endocarditis) infections. These infections, however, represent the minority of infections in cancer patients.

Bone marrow transplant, especially allogeneic (from a related donor), uses a special application of antimicrobial therapy. After the transplant, patients have persistent deficits in both humoral and cell-mediated immunity (Wingard 1990). During this time, the risk of infection is increased, and *pneumocystis carinii* pneumonia and cytomegalovirus infection are special concerns. The most commonly administered prophylactic therapies include initial aerosolized pentamidine followed by bactrim when blood count recovery is adequate, gamma globulin, and ganciclovir (Emmanuel et al. 1988; Pizzo et al. 1993; Wingard 1990).

Most chemotherapy is currently administered in the hospital (on in- and outpatient units) or in physicians' offices. For drugs (e.g., cisplatin) that require special hydration orders or monitoring for emesis or other side effects, these settings facilitate this process. For drugs that are given as an injection, an intravenous push, or a short infusion, the above-mentioned outpatient settings are most commonly employed, since they are generally convenient to the patient, can be combined with a planned patient visit or evaluation, and facilitate physician reimbursement for services rendered. The technology of high-tech home care is currently most useful for the administration of drugs that are given as a continuous infusion. The most common drug used in this manner is the antimetabolite 5-fluorouracil (Lokich et al. 1989). These infusions typically require central venous access and the use of an infusion pump. The availability of these technologies allows the patient to avoid inpatient hospitalization.

A special application of outpatient chemotherapy is used in the treatment of metastatic or primary liver disease (Blackshear et al. 1972; Kemeny et al. 1987). A catheter is placed surgically within the hepatic artery and is connected to a pump that is surgically implanted in the abdominal wall. This pump has a drug chamber and is driven by a charging fluid chamber. It can be accessed percutaneously and refilled every one to two weeks. These treatments are generally well tolerated, avoiding many of the customary systemic chemotherapy toxicities, delivering higher doses of drugs to the specific area of the tumor.

The administration of drugs and intravenous fluids at home is obviously not limited to the above examples. Established intravenous access and pump technology facilitates the administration of a variety of therapies either at home or in another ambulatory setting. Other examples are anticoagulation with heparin, the administration of blood products, amphotericin therapy for fungal infections, and intravenous fluids to prevent dehydration and treat hypercalcemia. Of course, as patients become more ill, many of these services may be best performed in a more supervised setting.

Respiratory Care

Shortness of breath is a common symptom in cancer patients. One study reported that 11 percent of patients with lung cancer referred for definitive radiation complained of dyspnea at presentation (Coy and Kennelly 1980). With disease progression, the frequency of dyspnea will increase.

The provision of oxygen supplementation in the home is well described by Pousada in chapter 7 of this volume. It should be emphasized that not all dyspnea in the cancer patient is best treated with supplemental oxygen. Shortness of breath in the cancer population is often multifactorial. Anemia, pleural/pericardial fluid, bronchitis/pneumonia, treatment toxicity (e.g., bleomycin), problems with secretions from a tracheostomy, and a misinterpreted complaint of fatigue or depression may be contributory and are more definitively treated by other means.

Tracheostomy care is commonly provided in the home. Appropriately sized catheters connected to a suction pump are used to help mobilize tracheal secretions. Local humidification prevents drying and facilitates the mobilization of these secretions. For patients with head and neck cancer, excessive oral secretions are often an issue, and appropriate suction helps them deal with this problem as well.

Mechanical ventilation, described at length by Okun in chapter 2 of this volume, is used on a selective basis, most commonly for patients with curable disease or a clearly reversible, self-limited problem. For patients with incurable progressive disease and a poor performance status, mechanical ventilatory support and other more aggressive and invasive resuscitative procedures are not encouraged, do little to alter the ultimate outcome, and can be deleterious to the quality of the patient's remaining life (Vitelli et al. 1991).

Benefits and Burdens of High-Tech Home Care

The most obvious benefit of high-tech home care for oncology patients is being able to maximize time at home. As Schachter and Holland note in chapter 6 of this volume, most patients prefer to be at home surrounded by family and friends. This is especially true for patients with incurable disease, where time at home will likely decrease as the disease progresses. Being at home allows patients to maintain greater independence and exert more control over their care. The patient is able to avoid exposure to various pathogens present in the hospital. The greater involvement of family members and caregivers in the management and support of the patient may have positive emotional effects on both the patient and caregiver and may facilitate emotional closure with a loved one who is dying. In theory, the costs are less for home services than for those provided in the hospital setting. (For a fuller account of problems associated with the cost of high-tech home care, see chap. 13.)

Despite the potential benefits of care in the home, there can be significant burdens affecting patients, families/caregivers, and involved medical professionals. Many potential benefits are linked to potential burdens, and are best viewed as challenges that must be effectively managed to deliver high-quality high-tech home care.

Although patients like the concept of being at home and closer to loved ones, they can miss the idea of being only a "call bell away" from the considerable expertise available in the hospital. For patients who are chronically ill with multiple comorbidities, a variety of symptoms are commonly present such that their anxiety and imagination can easily get the best of them.

Although professional backup and support are available, this is not the arena where high-tech home care companies make their profits. Unlike more traditional home care agencies, high-tech firms may market a service but make their profits on the various materials (e.g., intravenous fluids, drugs, pumps) used in the process of providing that service. The visiting health professional may not be the same for each visit and may not know the details of the patient's history first hand. Since visiting nurses are often responsible for multiple patients, the amount of time they can spend in each home is limited. Ill cancer patients often have multiple physical and emotional needs and need "high-touch" as much as, if not more than, "high-tech" care. These other needs are difficult if not impossible for the visiting nurse to address in the time available for a problem-focused home visit.

When in the home, the patient may become more detached from direct contact with the primary physician and staff. This patient-physician relationship can be an extremely important source of support for many patients. Providing "long distance" care is less professionally rewarding to the involved physician.

The provision of adequate home care depends on a supportive environment. While this can have a positive effect on relationships at home, it can also be a severe stress. Taking care of a chronically ill cancer patient will at times be exhausting and relentless for the caregiver. With a debilitated patient, the goal of self-administration is more of a challenge, the potential for treatment-related toxicity increases, and the dependence on a caregiver is greater. The risk exists that if an adverse event occurs, which for an ill or dying patient is often inevitable and perhaps increased in likelihood when technically sophisticated devices are monitored by a tired caregiver, the caregivers can easily blame themselves and feel guilty. If there are small children at home, they are able to see firsthand the illness and its effect on family relationships.

Although home care is less expensive than hospital-based care in absolute terms, the out-of-pocket cost to the patient may be more for the same service provided in the home, depending on the insurance coverage and the status (certified versus noncertified) of the home care company. For example, Medicare will currently cover the administration of only selected intravenous antibiotics in the home. There may also be hidden costs for physicians. Although the doctor may not see the patient as regularly, if at all, home care orders, disability and insurance forms, prescription renewals, and other paperwork are often still the responsibility of the primary physician. Adequate reimbursement for this often substantial investment of time can be difficult to obtain, especially when there is no actual visit for which to bill the patient.

The severity of illness for many of these patients can be quite significant, and defining stability for the purposes of home care is difficult. Cancer patients may be stable when originally discharged to the home, but their status can change quite rapidly. Furthermore, the goals of care for each patient (e.g., following bone marrow transplant vs. home hospice) are quite different. Depending on the situation, patients will have different monitoring requirements, and clinical deterioration will prompt different clinical decisions.

Many of the quality-assurance mechanisms now applied to care provided in more traditional settings are in the development and evolution stage for home care.

The entrepreneurial aspect of the home care industry will inevitably have an effect on its further development. There may be considerable financial pressures to expand into areas of expensive new technology in healthier patients with hopes of a higher profit margin, at the expense of the provision of other, less profitable but important services to those more ill. There is a receptive market for such thinking among cancer patients, as many individuals with incurable disease and limited therapeutic options are eager to gain access to new therapies even if their efficacy is unproven (Lerner and Kennedy 1992).

Future Directions

Fiscal pressures will increasingly influence the delivery of care to the cancer patient. It is likely that changes in the insurance reimbursement system will facilitate care at home and that the number of cancer patients supported in this manner will increase. The performance of reliable outcome studies formally documenting that services historically provided in the hospital can be delivered in the patient's home less expensively and without compromise in quality will be an important part of this process. Methods to alleviate and confront the burdens and challenges discussed above must be formulated to facilitate the most effective use of these services. High-tech home care companies not only will be involved with hospital discharges but also will compete on a larger scale for hospital admissions. There will be a need for the development of daytime infusion centers to facilitate the convenient outpatient administration of more complicated therapies in less-stable or otherwise less-supported patients. (The theme of alternative institutions for the delivery of high-tech home care is also addressed in chaps. 10 and 12.) More sophisticated communication systems will be developed to facilitate the close monitoring of services and perhaps decrease the need for home visits. A natural extension of this concept will be the development and use of pumps that can be programed or have changes made from a distance. The roles of physicians, nurses, and other health professionals will need to evolve to adjust to the delivery of this type of care in the home.

ACKNOWLEDGMENTS

I would like to thank the following individuals for their comments regarding different issues discussed in this manuscript: Dr. Daniel Coit (vascular access); Dr. Russell Portenoy (pain control); Dr. Moishe Shike (nutritional support); Dr. James Young (bone marrow transplant); Karen Londa (social work); Joann Marcucci (nursing); Sharad Madison and William Slattery (high-tech home care industry).

REFERENCES

Aisner, J., Paines, H., Tait, N., et al. 1990. Appetite stimulation and weight gain with megestrol acetate. *Seminars in Oncology* 17 (suppl. 9):2–7.
Blackshear, P. J., Dorman, F. D., Blackshear, P. L., Jr., et al. 1972. The design and initial testing of an implantable infusion pump. *Surgery, Gynecology and Obstetrics* 134:51–56.
Boring, C. C., Squires, T. S., and Tong, T. 1991. Cancer statistics, 1991. *CA: A Cancer Journal for Clinicians* 41:19–36.
Bruera, E., Brenneis, C., Perry, B., and MacDonald, R. N. 1987. *Continuous subcutaneous administration of narcotics for the treatment of cancer pain.* Markham, Ont.: KNOLL Pharmaceuticals Canada.
Cherny, N. I., and Portenoy R. K. 1993. Cancer pain management: Current strategy. *Cancer* 72 (suppl.):3393–3415.
Clark, G. M., Sledge, G. W., Jr., Osborne, K. C., and McGuire, W. L. 1986. Survival from first recurrence: Relative importance of prognostic factors in 1,015 breast cancer patients. *Journal of Clinical Oncology* 4:1162–70.
Coy, P., and Kennelly, G. M. 1980. The role of curative radiotherapy in the treatment of lung cancer. *Cancer* 45:698–702.
Coyle, N., Monzillo, E., Loscalzo, M., Farkas, C., Massie, M. J., and Foley, K. M. 1985. A model of continuity of care for cancer patients with pain and neuro-oncologic complications. *Cancer Nursing* 8:111–19.
Crawford, E. D., Eisenberger, M. A., McLeod, D. G., et al. 1989. A controlled trial of leuprolide with and without flutamide in prostatic carcinoma. *New England Journal of Medicine* 321:419–24.
DeVita, V. T., Jr. 1990. The problem of resistance. *PPO Updates* 4:1–12.
DeWys, W. D., Begg, C., Lavin, P. T., et al. 1980. Prognostic effect of weight loss prior to chemotherapy in cancer patients. *American Journal of Medicine* 69:491–500.
Emmanuel, D., Cunningham, I., Jules-Elysee, K., et al. 1988. Cytomegalovirus pneumonia after bone marrow transplantation successfully treated with the combination of ganciclovir and high-dose intravenous immune globulin. *Annals of Internal Medicine* 109:777–83.

Groeger, J. S., Lucas, A. B., and Coit, D. 1991. Venous access in the cancer patient. *PPO Updates* 5:1–14.

Groth-Juncker, A., and McCusker, J. 1983. Where do elderly patients prefer to die? *Journal of the American Geriatrics Society* 31:457–61.

Kemeny, N., Daly, J., Reichman, B., et al. 1987. Intrahepatic or systemic infusion of fluorodeoxyuridine in patients with liver metastasis from colorectal carcinoma. *Annals of Internal Medicine* 107:459–65.

Kennedy, B. J. 1992. *Aging and Cancer*. ASCO Educational Book, p. 250. Chicago: American Society of Clinical Oncology.

Lerner, I. J., and Kennedy, B. J. 1992. The prevalence of questionable methods of cancer treatment in the United States. *CA: A Cancer Journal for Clinicians* 42:181–91.

Lokich, J. J., Ahlgren, J. D., Gullo, J. J., et al. 1989. A prospective randomized comparison of continuous infusion fluorouracil with conventional bolus schedule in metastatic colorectal carcinoma: A Mid-Atlantic Oncology Program study. *Journal of Clinical Oncology* 7:425–32.

Pizzo, P. A., Myers, J., Freifeld, A. G., and Walsh, T. 1993. Infections in the cancer patient. In V. T. DeVita, Jr., S. Hellman, and S. A. Rosenberg, eds., *Cancer: Principles and Practice of Oncology*, 4th ed., pp. 2292–2337. Philadelphia: J. B. Lippincott.

Portenoy, R. K. 1989. Cancer pain: Epidemiology and syndromes. *Cancer* 63 (suppl.):2298–2307.

Rubenstein, E. B., Rolston, K., Benjamin, R. S., et al. 1993. *Cancer* 71:3640–46.

Shike, M. 1992. Nutritional support of the cancer patient. *Triangle* 31:25–33.

Shike, M., Berner, Y. N., Gerdes, H., et al. 1989. Percutaneous endoscopic gastrostomy and jejunostomy for long-term feeding in patients with cancer of the head and neck. *Otolaryngology—Head and Neck Surgery* 101:549–54.

Tuyns, A. J. 1982. Alcohol. In D. Schottenfeld and J. F. Fraumeni, eds., *Cancer Epidemiology and Prevention*, pp. 293–303. Philadelphia: W. B. Saunders.

Vitelli, C. E., Cooper, K., Rogatko, A., and Brennan, M. F. 1991. Cardiopulmonary resuscitation in the patient with cancer. *Journal of Clinical Oncology* 9:111–15.

Wingard, J. R. 1990. Management of infectious complications of bone marrow transplantation. *Oncology* 4:69–75.

Wynder, E. L., and Hoffmann, D. 1982. Tobacco. In D. Schottenfeld and J. F. Fraumeni, eds., *Cancer Epidemiology and Prevention*, pp. 277–92. Philadelphia: W. B. Saunders.

5. Issues in Long-Term and High-Tech Home Care for Persons with HIV Infection/AIDS

Angela McCabe, C.S.W., Josephine Paredes, M.D., and David G. Pfister, M.D.

In 1981, several investigators reported infections that typically occur in patients with compromised immune resistance (so-called opportunistic infections), a rare cancer (Kaposi sarcoma [KS]), or both, in an epidemiologically restricted population (CDC 1981; Gottlieb et al. 1981). This illness, characterized by profound immune defects, was eventually termed acquired immune-deficiency syndrome (AIDS) and was found to be caused by infection with a newly recognized human retrovirus, now termed human immunodeficiency virus (HIV). Initially cases were reported in sexually active homosexual males and intravenous drug users. Individuals who received blood transfusions or blood-component therapy, children born to mothers who were intravenous drug users, prostitutes, and sexual partners of bisexual males and drug users were later identified as having similar defects and clinical manifestations (CDC 1987). Since the initial recognition of the syndrome, persons with AIDS have been diagnosed in all inhabited continents.

HIV disease represents a spectrum of illness. The clinical evolution follows the progression of the viral disease and associated destruction of a certain blood cell subset (CD4+ T-lymphocytes) (CDC 1992), leading to increasing immune deficiency and progressive clinical disease. The use of medical care, including high-tech and other home care services, depends on the stage of infection afflicting a patient.

After primary infection, an HIV-positive patient enters a pro-

79

longed period whose duration is impossible to predict, called the asymptomatic carrier stage. Some patients are not completely asymptomatic, in that they may have persistent generalized lymphadenopathy, also known as AIDS-related complex (ARC), but even in these cases the patient's level of function generally is excellent and the health care requirements minimal. After this stage, however, the patient may begin to show symptoms of progressive viral disease and immune deficiency, such as unexplained and prolonged fevers, involuntary weight loss, profuse night sweats, and prolonged diarrhea. This period may be marked by a number of infections that are often tenacious, such as oral candidiasis (thrush), and by increasing neurological manifestations.

AIDS, which requires a current or past history of an opportunistic infection or immune deficiency-related cancer, is the end stage of HIV disease. The opportunistic infections that can occur commonly involve the lungs (e.g., bacterial infections, *Pneumocystis carinii* pneumonia [PCP], tuberculosis, atypical mycobacteriosis), eyes (e.g., cytomegalovirus [CMV], toxoplasmosis), gastrointestinal tract (e.g., *Cryptosporidium*, isosporiasis, candidiasis, CMV), and central nervous system (e.g., toxoplasmosis, cryptococcosis, HIV encephalopathy). The cancers that occur most commonly are KS and certain types of lymphoma (CDC 1992). Any of these AIDS-related illnesses can ultimately lead to the patient's demise. The clinical course is characterized by progressive deterioration and debilitation and, depending on the site of involvement, more specific morbidities such as blindness and dementia.

Individuals diagnosed with AIDS first focus on the current medical crisis. Only when the acute symptoms diminish are they able to confront the reality and experience the emotional impact of the diagnosis. Individuals are confronted with their own mortality, fears of physical debilitation, neurological impairment, and loss of independence, and each successive hospitalization is a reminder of the disease and its consequences. Most of the AIDS-defining opportunistic infections currently require an acute hospital admission. The availability of various high-tech home care services facilitates complicated care in the outpatient/home setting and thus can decrease the length of stay and hospitalization rate, decrease the emotional impact of repeated hospitalization, and enhance the quality of life for these patients.

Between 1 million and 1.5 million Americans are infected with HIV; to date, only 10 percent of those infected have been diagnosed with AIDS. As HIV progresses in this population, new HIV infections occur, new cases of AIDS are diagnosed, and their longevity increases; health care needs including high-tech services will continue to increase dramatically. Providing medical care to persons with HIV/ AIDS represents a tremendous challenge and involves significant medical, psychological, and social issues.

Medical Management

The medical management of HIV infection focuses on two major goals: delay in the progression of HIV infection to AIDS and improvement in the quality and length of life for persons who have progressed to an AIDS diagnosis. Many interventions require high-tech support.

Antiretroviral Therapy

At present, zidovudine (AZT), didanosine (ddI), zalcitabine (ddC), and zerit (D4T) are the only specific antiretroviral therapies formally approved for HIV infection, and all are generally administered orally (Fischl et al. 1987, 1990; Yarchoan et al. 1988, 1990). AZT is recommended for patients with HIV infection with fewer than 500 CD4 cells/mm^3. There is evidence that AZT can increase survival when administered to symptomatic HIV-infected patients with fewer than 200 CD4 cells/mm^3, and that short-term progression to AIDS or severe ARC can be decreased by the administration of AZT to patients with 200 to 500 CD4 cells/mm^3. DdI, ddC, and D4T are used for patients who cannot tolerate or who have failed AZT therapy. Given the limitations of current antiretrovial therapy, many patients participate in clinical trials of new drugs.

Treatment of HIV-Related Complications

All patients with progressive HIV infection anticipate a series of complications because of their immune compromise. Treatment may be preventive in patients identified as at high risk for a given complication, or it may begin after the complication has occurred. Intravenous therapy is often necessary. If the patient is clinically stable, many of the subsequently described treatments can be administered in the ambulatory/home setting when high-tech services are available. The therapies often require ongoing venous access, which is best provided by some type of chronic indwelling central venous catheter, as described by Pfister in Chapter 4, this volume.

Preventive Treatment. The most common AIDS-defining complication in persons with HIV infection is PCP. Persons with CD4 lymphocyte counts below 200/mm^3, CD4 percentage below 20, early symptoms and signs of HIV infection, and a previous history of PCP are at highest risk for PCP (Masur et al. 1989). Consequently, PCP prophylaxis, generally with oral trimethoprim-sulfamethoxazole or aerosolized pentamidine (as in bone marrow transplant patients), is now recommended for these patients. Randomized data suggest that the former is more effective, although it can be associated with more side effects (Schneider et al. 1992). Preventive treatment is being explored for tuberculosis and other mycobacterial infections, toxoplasmosis, and fungal and CMV infections.

Acute and Chronic Treatment of Infection. Many infections are widely disseminated at the time of diagnosis and are prone to relapse, given the patient's compromised immune status. Thus, after initial treatment of the infection, ongoing chronic suppressive therapy is required to decrease the morbidity of repeated infections. As the number of infectious complications increases, so does the complexity of an individual's chronic suppressive treatment, making timely administration of the appropriate regimens in the home setting increasingly difficult. Examples of this increasing complexity include the use of intravenous amphotericin B for induction therapy of cryptococcal meningitis or candidiasis resistant to oral antifungal therapy; intravenous gancyclovir or foscarnet for the treatment of CMV retinitis; intravenous pentamidine for the treatment of PCP; and intravenous amikacin for the treatment of active *Mycobacterium avium-intracellulare* (MAI) infection. With improved recognition of infectious complications, improved treatment options for these complications, and the use of survival-prolonging antiretroviral drugs, many persons with AIDS are now developing multiple chronic infections that necessitate lifelong suppression (CDC 1992).

The neurological complications of HIV infection are also relatively common. Among the most problematic are HIV-associated peripheral neuropathy and dementia. These neurocognitive and behavioral abnormalities may respond to therapy with AZT (Navia, Jordan, and Price 1986; Price and Brew, 1990).

Treatment of Malignancies. The growing list of options for the treatment or prevention of opportunistic infections and the suppression of the underlying HIV infection often makes it necessary to modify antineoplastic treatments to accommodate other therapies and preventive strategies.

KS is often initially superficial, progresses slowly, and is treated on an outpatient basis. Although most, if not all, of the clinical manifestations of KS are not directly life threatening, they may be associated with significant physical disability. For example, extensive swelling, particularly of the lower extremities, may be associated with ulceration of cutaneous lesions, serous drainage, and bacterial superinfection, requiring daily skin care and topical, oral, or intravenous antibacterial therapy. Some lesions, particularly those on the feet, may be painful and require oral or parenteral narcotics for symptom relief. In addition, the disfiguring lesions present a major source of isolation and rejection, and even a few lesions may serve as a constant reminder of the illness. The three early treatment approaches—chemotherapy, radiation therapy, and so-called biological therapy with interferon-α—remain the core of the therapeutic armamentarium today, and most are administered intravenously or subcutaneously. Locally symptomatic disease may respond to radiation therapy (Krown, Myskowski, and Paredes 1992).

Non-Hodgkin lymphomas also occur in persons with HIV infection. Primary treatment options include chemotherapy and radiation therapy (Levine 1992).

The use of proteins that stimulate certain components of the bone marrow (so-called hematopoietic growth factors) has expanded to prevent treatment-induced bone marrow suppression in HIV-infected patients. These medicines are generally administered subcutaneously, although they can be administered intravenously. Granulocyte colony-stimulating factor (G-CSF) and granulocyte-macrophage colony-stimulating factor (GM-CSF) ameliorate disease or treatment-related depressions in the white blood count. In addition, erythropoietin, which is also administered subcutaneously, has markedly reduced the requirements for red blood cell transfusion, primarily in patients with pretreatment serum erythropoietin levels below 500 mμ/ml (Sieff 1990).

Pain Management. Patients with HIV/AIDS often experience acute and chronic pain. Inadequate pain control may decrease the patient's activity. This inactivity can cause additional problems, such as muscle atrophy, gastrointestinal and pulmonary complications, and emotional despair.

Pain management and the potential role for high-tech home care services are well described by Pfister in chapter 4 of this volume. One of the factors complicating pain management in some patients is a history of drug abuse. At times families, partners, and physicians tend to resist the use of pain medication and frequently do not believe the patient's complaints. They are often suspicious of the reported pain and are fearful of the patient's return to drug use and dependency. Pain medications can have cross-tolerance with addictive substances. The patient's anxiety will increase when pain and physical deterioration are complicated by these and related issues.

Hydration and Nutrition. Many patients with AIDS will have inadequate fluid and nutritional intake. The potential causes are multiple, including treatment-related side effects, disease or infection involving the oral cavity and/or esophagus, chronic diarrhea, neurological impairment, and general debilitation. When possible, hydration and nutritional needs are managed through the existing gastrointestinal tract rather than intravenously. This approach costs less and is associated with less morbidity. A nasogastric feeding tube or feeding gastrostomy/jejunostomy will often be needed to facilitate this process if the problem is chronic.

Intravenous hydration can be provided through either a peripheral or a central vein. It should be emphasized that typical intravenous fluids replace fluids and electrolytes but are not an adequate source of complete nutrition.

Total parenteral nutrition (TPN) typically requires central venous access for administration. It is expensive and can lead to significant metabolic abnormalities if administered without appropriate monitoring. TPN should be used judiciously, with a focus on those patients for whom it will produce major benefits.

Home parenteral nutrition (HPN) is a relatively new therapy. A number of large academic centers have reported their experience with HPN and have described successful rehabilitation of patients with a variety of benign diseases causing short bowel syndrome. These early positive reports encouraged more widespread use of the therapy, and in recent years it has expanded to involve more short-term clinical situations, including patients with neoplastic bowel obstruction or cachexia (extreme weight loss) associated with AIDS. Despite intuitive impressions that HPN should reduce mortality and improve organ function in patients with AIDS, the results from clinical studies have not been conclusive. There is little published scientific evidence to support the routine use of HPN in AIDS patients with serious continuing systemic disease. An analysis of the United Kingdom's HPN registry fails to demonstrate that such patients benefit from this treatment (Mughal et al. 1986). Several studies have shown that the best results from HPN are seen in patients in whom primary intestinal failure is the cause of malnutrition. In a study by Kotler et al. (1990), the AIDS patients who showed benefit were those for whom malabsorption was the principal factor for the weight loss.

Home Care Issues

Psychosocial Issues

With fears of disease progression, individuals often feel pressured to disclose their diagnosis to family and friends. Fears of rejection, panic, and sadness often affect their ability to communicate with the people closest to them. This causes further isolation and loneliness. Prior life choices may have led many patients to distance themselves from their families. Since much high-tech home care requires an involved family member or caregiver, especially when the patient becomes progressively debilitated, social isolation can limit high-tech options. One of the goals of supportive counseling is to continue the process of diminishing social isolation through helping the patient disclose information to the appropriate individual(s) and agencies who can provide ongoing support. It is important to secure both formal and informal supports for the patient. This will help sustain the patient through acute medical episodes, including treatment failures.

Patients fear the social impact of AIDS and their dependency on family, friends, colleagues, and staff. Since persons with AIDS are generally a young population, they become concerned about being a burden and how others will respond: will their caregivers get tired of helping, abandon or reject them, or become uncomfortable and not know what to say? They feel less valuable because they are unable to be productive, while concurrently draining their social and financial resources.

Caregivers are confused when they feel the need to withdraw or run away or want the person to die and be released from intense suffering, while simultaneously feeling an urgency to ensure that the patient does not die alone. This ambivalence can be exacerbated in relationships in which there are previously unresolved problems or extraordinary anger and fears of abandonment. The stress on caregivers is especially difficult when they are solely responsible for high-tech and other home care. As the illness progresses, the stress on the caregiver and the complexity of care increase, as does the potential for mistakes. Errors can affect the patient, but can also endanger the caregiver. Accidental sticks with an intravenous needle, for example, pose a risk of HIV infection.

Assisting the patient in planning for surviving members is very important. Although the successful completion of each task may involve underlying thoughts of impending separation, it can bring about a sense of resolution and completion. Typical tasks include making a will, contacting family members, working through value differences, discussing financial affairs, and prearranging a funeral. Additional problems concern repairing estranged relationships, arranging foster care and adoption for children, and ensuring that appropriate benefits go to the common-law wife/lover. Patients often experience tremendous relief on the completion of these tasks and often exhibit an increased ability to share their feelings and thoughts about the dying process.

Mental health care providers need to provide grief counseling and bereavement services to the survivors of people with AIDS. These individuals fear a loss of income, lack of emotional support, alienation, and physical and social abuse, and often feel their options for future relationships are limited.

Discharge Planning

Home care needs are explored and identified by the physician, nurse, social worker, patient, family, friends, insurance case manager, and community service providers. By providing a safe plan, it is hoped that the patient will be discharged from the hospital with diminished feelings of hopelessness and helplessness. The assessment must take into account the patient's physical and emotional frailty, possible symptoms of dementia, or other significant morbidities such as blindness, and evaluate environmental resources involving finances, housing, and insurance. An assessment of the family or friends' willingness and/or capacity to provide adequate care or to learn the necessary skills is vital. The strength of the individual's social supports becomes an increasingly important factor in assessing a patient's capacity to cope with future stresses as the illness progresses and to determine the feasibility of various home care options. Unfortunately, the necessary home care is often not reimbursable because of insurance limitations, posing a significant barrier to successful discharge planning (see Insurance section below).

HIV/AIDS can affect patients from a wide variety of socioeconomic backgrounds, and this has obvious implications for discharge planning and the delivery of high-tech home care services. Recent trends suggest that while the proportion of HIV/AIDS cases in homosexual and bisexual men has slowly decreased, the number of cases among intravenous drug abusers and their sexual partners has increased (CDC 1993). Many of these latter individuals live in extremely impoverished home situations. Some are homeless, living in shelters, on the streets, or rotating nights among various friends, family, or other acquaintances. For others, the available housing is often small, poorly maintained, furnished with limited and/or outdated household appliances, and located in high-crime areas. Problems with sanitation, bugs, and rodents are common. Many of the patients are alone or isolated, while others live in grossly overcrowded conditions. Identifying a responsible and committed caregiver is often a problem. Medical supplies such as needles, syringes, and narcotics are at risk for being stolen, and in the event of an equipment failure or other problem, the safety and security of the visiting high-tech home care nurse or technician is a major concern. Faced with these potential obstacles, all but the simplest outpatient regimens are difficult, if not impossible, to orchestrate.

The limited availability of social support, home care services, and the community support services for patients, partners, families, and friends adds to the difficulty in delivering effective treatment and providing adequate outpatient services. In New York City, which has the largest HIV population in the United States, few chronic and terminal beds or supervised living residencies are willing to accept these patients. Therefore, many patients are forced to stay in the hospital even though supervised home care would be sufficient and would provide a better quality of life. A continuum of care including acute care facilities, supervised living, chronic or nursing home, and hospice care is required in every community (see chaps. 10 and 12, this volume). To meet the changing medical and social needs of these individuals with AIDS, easy access to facilities and flexibility in moving to different levels of care are needed.

High-Tech Services

A growing number of providers have developed specialized home care programs for people with AIDS. These programs have been developed to meet the patients' needs as advances in technology enable more sophisticated care to be offered in home settings. Some of the common treatments administered in the home include antibiotic infusion therapy (e.g., antibacterial, antifungal, and antiviral), chemotherapy, blood transfusions, pain management, venipuncture and central line insertion, respiratory care, nebulizer treatments, aerosolized pentamidine therapy for PCP prophylaxis, tube feedings for enteral nutrition therapy, and intravenous hydration. Nursing visits are also required to assist patients with the care of a central venous catheter (dressing changes and periodic flushing with anticoagulant to prevent the catheter from clotting), subcutaneous injections (e.g., interferon-α therapy, hematopoietic growth factors such as G-CSF and/or erythropoietin), wound care and dressing changes (sterile, nonsterile), aggressive skin care (soaks to infected Kaposi lesions, decubiti [bed sores], superficial fungal or viral infections), and monitoring of vital signs.

The high-tech home care needs of AIDS patients are often extensive and complicated. The agenda for a nursing visit can be so full that little time is left to address important emotional issues (Schachter and Holland, chap. 6, below). Home visit responsibilities will often rotate among several different nurses, further compounding the problem. This limitation underscores the important role of the primary caregiver.

Insurance Issues

Life and health insurance are very important to people with HIV/AIDS but can present many challenging problems to both the patient and the provider. Major barriers to affordable health insurance include (*a*) refusal of new applications; (*b*) policy reductions and cancellations; (*c*) higher premiums when converting from group to individual policies; (*d*) denial due to pre-existing condition; and (*e*) extended waiting periods. Without insurance, these individuals are left with the choice of bankruptcy in the event of catastrophic illness or "spending down" to the poverty level to be eligible for state Medicaid benefits.

Most patients with HIV conditions receive professional care at home. Many live alone, some with families or friends. Because of the regulatory provisions of Medicaid, Medicare, Blue Cross/Blue Shield, and many other insurers and health maintenance organizations, a certified home health care agency (e.g., Visiting Nurse Service) must be used for home care services. Very few insurance companies reimburse services to proprietary nursing agencies. While the care demands on family and friends are enormous, few respite services or resources are provided for them.

Summary

Until all patients' needs can be adequately addressed, we need to be creative in expanding the current programs in the community and in developing new programs that can continue to serve the growing needs of patients with HIV/AIDS, their families, and their friends. High-tech home care can be an important part of this process, but it is clearly only one aspect of any comprehensive outpatient care program. As previously discussed, insurance problems, patient debilitation, and social isolation can make high-tech home care planning especially challenging for these patients.

REFERENCES

Centers for Disease Control (CDC). 1981. Kaposi's sarcoma and pneumocystis among homosexual men, New York and California. *Morbidity and Mortality Weekly Report* 30:305.

———. 1987. Revision of the CDC surveillance case definition for acquired immunodeficiency syndrome. *Morbidity and Mortality Weekly Report* 36 (suppl. 1S):3S-14S.

———. 1992. 1993 revised classification system for HIV infection and expanded surveillance case definition for AIDS among adolescents and adults. *Morbidity and Mortality Weekly Report* (Recommendations and Reports RR-17) 41:1–19.

———. 1993. *HIV/AIDS Surveillance Report.*

Fischl, M. A., Richman, D. D., Grieco, M. H., et al. 1987. The efficacy of azidothymidine (AZT) in the treatment of patients with AIDS and AIDS-related complex: A double-blind, placebo-controlled trial. *New England Journal of Medicine* 317:185–91.

Fischl, M. A., Richman, D. D., Hansen, N., et al. 1990. The safety and efficacy of zidovudine (AZT) in the treatment of subjects with mildly symptomatic human immunodeficiency virus type I (HIV) infection: A double-blind, placebo-controlled trial. *Annals of Internal Medicine* 112:727–37.

Gottlieb, M. S., Schroff, R., Schanker, H. M., et al. 1981. Pneumocystis carinii pneumonia and mucosal candidiasis in previously healthy homosexual men. Evidence of a new acquired cellular immunodeficiency. *New England Journal of Medicine* 305:1425–31.

Kotler, D. P., Tierney, A. R., Culpepper-Morgan, J. A., et al. 1990. Effect of home total parenteral nutrition on body composition in patients with acquired immunodeficiency syndrome. *Journal of Parenteral Nutrition* 14:454–58.

Krown, S. E., Myskowski, P. L., and Paredes, J. 1992. Kaposi's sarcoma. *Medical Clinics of North America* 76:235–52.

Levine, A. M. 1992. AIDS-associated malignant lymphoma. *Medical Clinics of North America* 76:253–68.

Masur, H., Ognibene, F. P., Yarchoan, R., et al. 1989. CD4 counts as predictors of opportunistic pneumonias in human immunodeficiency virus (HIV) infection. *Annals of Internal Medicine* 111:223–31.

Mughal, M., Irving, M., on behalf of U.K. Home Parenteral Nutrition Group. 1986. Home parenteral nutrition in the United Kingdom and Ireland. *Lancet* ii:383–87.

Navia, B. A., Jordon, B. D., and Price, R. W. 1986. The AIDS dementia complex: I. Clinical features. *Annals of Neurology* 19:517–24.

Price, R. W., and Brew, B. 1990. Management of the neurologic complications of HIV-1 infection and AIDS. In M. A. Sande and P. A. Volberding, eds., *The Medical Management of AIDS*, pp. 161–81. Philadelphia: W. B. Saunders.

Schneider, M. M., Hoepelman, A. I. M., Eeftinck Schattenkerk, J. K. M., et al. 1992. A controlled trial of aerosolized pentamidine or trimethoprim-sulfamethoxazole as primary prophylaxis against pneumocystis carinii pneumonia in patients with human immunodeficiency virus infection. *New England Journal of Medicine* 327:1836–41.

Sieff, C. A. 1990. Biology and clinical aspects of the hematopoietic growth factors. *Annual Review of Medicine* 41:483–96.

Yarchoan, R., Perno, C. F., Thomas, R. V., et al. 1988. Phase I studies of 2′,3′-dideoxycytidine in severe human immunodeficiency virus infection as a single agent and alternating with zidovudine (AZT). *Lancet* i:76–81.

Yarchoan, R., Pluda, J. M., Thomas, R. V., et al. 1990. Long-term toxicity/activity profile of 2′,3′-dideoxyinosine in AIDS or AIDS-related complex. *Lancet* 336:526–29.

6. Psychological, Social, and Ethical Issues in the Home Care of Terminally Ill Patients

THE IMPACT OF TECHNOLOGY

Sherry R. Schachter, R.N., M.A.,
and Jimmie C. Holland, M.D.

Home is where most individuals prefer to be when they are ill, especially when the illness is serious. This desire becomes stronger when the illness is chronic, or when it is progressive and likely to be fatal. Until recently, however, home care of chronic and terminal illness was limited because only the most basic medical care could be given there; in addition, the medical team did not regard family members and caregivers as partners in caring for the patient. The hospice movement started in this country in the 1960s and began to encourage families to assume a more central role in the care of their dying relatives. Previously, the hospital was the major alternative, where too often terminal care became impersonal and insensitive. The hospice model displayed the integration of care at home by the family. This model provided the use of special inpatient beds when needed. Care was then given by a staff trained in the management of the physical, psychological, and spiritual needs of dying people. Hospice programs had the disadvantage of sometimes not being closely related to the patient's medical care. This required a new team of hospice caregivers that replaced the patient's familiar physician and staff at a particularly difficult time for the patient and family.

The 1990s has seen drastic changes in patterns of care in which the major responsibility for patients has shifted from institutions back to the family; home is where more care is given for longer periods. Driven by economics, patients are being sent home from hospitals "sicker and quicker." They receive care that includes the use of highly technical equipment. In earlier days the high-tech care would have been applied only in the hospital by highly trained staff. Family caregivers have suddenly become paramount in home care. They are enlisted and instructed in the management of the machines placed in the home and are expected to administer complicated treatments on a rigid schedule. Since the broad definition of "family" includes individuals with whom the patient has a consistent and enduring relationship, close friends or relatives often become the primary caretakers.

The technology for delivering antibiotics, blood products, parenteral nutrition, and analgesia by infusion pumps and feeding tubes has provided the opportunity for many more patients to be treated and managed at home. The complexities of equipment require expert technical advice to assure their proper use at home. Home health agencies began to proliferate rapidly, providing a new, highly profitable arena for economic expansion. These agencies have not yet been examined by regulatory agencies for their profit margin. (See chap. 13, below.) Irrespective of the reason, the high cost of care at home can often exceed the cost for the same care in the hospital. Using the example of total parenteral nutrition, Arno et al. describe the huge disparity between the charges to the patient at home and the actual costs to the agency providing the services.

Recently, the home has emerged as a more viable option for patients with chronic and terminal illness (Bergen 1992; Ferrell et al. 1991; Grobe, Ilstrup, and Ahmann 1981; Hileman, Lackey, and Hassanein 1992; Sankar, 1991; Siegel et al., 1991). It is, therefore, an appropriate time to assess the impact of the home care option for dying patients and their families. The cost to families has clearly not been addressed in the policy arena, yet the cost for full-time paid caregivers at home can run from $25,000 to $40,000 per year. The cost of an infusion pump to deliver patient-controlled analgesia (PCA), for example, can easily add $100 per day. It has been estimated that in 1992, 2.7 million adult children in the United States provided unpaid care for elderly parents. Health care policy and reform must examine the cost and extent of home care services for both chronic and terminal illness, their values, and their abuse for profit.

Another critically important social change that affects the care of terminal illness at home is the public debate regarding physician-assisted suicide and euthanasia. Frail, elderly patients who are depressed are more vulnerable to feelings of being an economic and physical burden. They are more apt to request hastened death, as they perceive that they are causing fatigue and distress to their loved ones who are the caregivers. The current social debate has had the effect of increasing patients' requests for physician-assisted suicide by terminally ill individuals. Yet, when these individuals' distress, depression, or pain is effectively controlled by interventions applied at home, they are willing to spend their remaining time with loved ones.

While the technology now available and employed at home is similar in its application for use in both chronic and terminal illness, the goals, time frame, and illness trajectory are quite different. This chapter presents the issues as they relate to terminal illness, outlining the goals, benefits, liabilities, and clinical issues. We make several recommendations that support our position that patients with terminal-stage illness can be managed successfully and sensitively at home. We emphasize that aggressive use of high technology at home for palliative care is appropriate for symptom control.

The Goals of Terminal Care at Home

The goal of terminal care at home should be to provide medical and psychosocial care directed toward maximal comfort, quality of life, and psychological well-being. Despite advancing illness, the technology available at home today substantially enhances the potential for maintaining comfort. However, the same technology can be used with the wrong goals in mind. Advanced technological equipment may be applied for a longer period than is appropriate, which can interfere with the goal of maximal comfort. Our recommendation about high-tech interventions is simple: they should be introduced to meet specific, identified needs for enhancing patient/family comfort that cannot be met by a simpler means.

In addition, the medical status of patients receiving palliative care is constantly changing. It is important to monitor high-tech interventions for their appropriateness so that they are continued for only as long as they are meeting the need for which they were introduced. They should be withdrawn when they no longer contribute to the patient's comfort or quality of life.

The specific high-tech measures discussed in this chapter are those most often deployed in terminal care: oxygen; infusion pumps for analgesia; parenteral and feeding devices; and venous access for giving blood, blood products, and antibiotics. (See chap. 4, this volume, for details.)

Making the Decision for Home Care

The first issue in successful home care is to determine if patients and family caregivers understand the obligations that home care will entail and whether they will learn to use the medical equipment and give treatments as prescribed. Successful home care also requires a simultaneous evaluation of the family by the physician or nurse, as to the family's motivation, psychological strengths and weaknesses, and reasonable expectations and the needed social and economic resources available to them. Coyle, Loscalzo, and Bailey (1990) developed a classification of families, based on these aspects and their ability to manage a loved one at home. Group 1 is comprised of families who will probably succeed in home care: they exhibit positive psychological strengths, have a history of good coping mechanisms, and have a support system that can be called on besides the immediate family. An evaluation of the patients' financial resources and/or independent health care coverage is essential at the outset to determine the feasibility of meeting the potentially prohibitive costs of home health aides, nurses, and medical equipment.

The individuals in group 2 have some negative qualities but will be able to manage with good home care support. Additionally, even families in group 1 may become fatigued over time and develop chronic stress that may lead them to seek more help.

Group 3, by contrast, consists of families in which either the patient or a caregiver has a history of psychiatric disturbance, such as alcoholism or substance abuse, or there is serious conflict. They may have unrealistic expectations of outcome, have poor social ties and support, and lack sufficient economic resources or insurance coverage. These families require extensive resources to succeed with home care. The Psychiatry Service Home Care Program at Memorial Sloan-Kettering Cancer Center is such a resource. Its goal is to assist families who may, by virtue of illness complications or prior psychological problems, require assistance in coping with the death of a loved one. The cornerstone of the program is the nurse clinician who is skilled in cancer nursing, pain management, and psychological issues. The nurse serves as liaison by twenty-four-hour beeper call, backed up by the psychiatric staff.

These three categories are useful in developing a home care plan that sets realistic goals with the patient and family. Additionally, it is important to recognize that the staff can also become stressed by the demands of managing difficult families at home. It is not only helpful but also essential that they too recognize those families who will pose more management problems and hence can have greater thought put into their care plan to anticipate the issues likely to arise.

Home care for the dying patient is not a feasible option for all families. Each situation must be carefully examined to determine its safety and appropriateness in maintaining the patient's optimal quality of life. This initial evaluation is conducted by an oncology nurse whose professional skills should include (a) the management of psychological and medical complications, (b) recognition of the influence and importance of family dynamics, (c) knowledge about medical and psychological issues in dying, and (d) proficiency in bereavement counseling. When the nurse determines that home care is not a reasonable option for a particular family, it is inappropriate to exert pressure on or blame the family (Schachter 1992).

Once the decision is made to undertake a home care plan, the health professional must intervene effectively and support the patient and the primary caregiver, who are viewed as a unit of care. The role that the family assumes in caring for the patient depends on their level of education in giving care and managing complex equipment and on the physical and emotional needs that change with the progression of disease. This leads to a dynamic relationship between the dying patient and the family, which contributes to the stresses imposed on the family structure.

Physical, Psychological, and Social Consequences

Many studies have identified the management of the patient's physical symptoms as the most difficult aspect of home care (Grobe, Ilstrup, and Ahmann 1981). Brown, Davies, and Martens (1990) reported physical problems as the major focus of stress. This stress was increased for the caregiver by the demands of giving nursing care without medical knowledge or nursing skills. The most stressful physical symptom to manage is pain, which is present in 60 to 90 percent of patients dying of cancer (Coyle 1989). The distress of seeing a loved one in pain can be difficult, and management, even in the most skilled hands, may require considerable titration of medications. Ferrell and co-workers (1991) noted the distress for both patient and caregiver. On the one hand, the caregiver fears giving too much medication, reducing the level of alertness, oversedating the person, or even hastening death. On the other hand, the caregiver fears giving too little medication and leaving the patient in pain. Self-doubt and guilt are common in the caregiver at such a time. In fact, inadequate pain control was observed by Brown, Davies, and Martens (1990) as the primary reason for the rehospitalization of home care patients. (McCabe, Paredes, and Pfister discuss routes of administering pain management in chapter 5 of this volume.) As the disease progresses, oral administration, the most preferred route, may no longer be feasible, and patients will require parenteral drugs to control their pain (see chap. 4, this volume). Families often describe PCA pumps as being too confusing and difficult to operate.

Other troublesome and common symptoms to manage at home are shortness of breath, weakness, anorexia, and constipation. The control of these symptoms may be difficult, but efforts to do so are critical for the patient to sense that the caregiver is trying; even partial success is reassuring. The following case exemplifies the important role of educating and instructing family members in the home management of cancer pain.

Case Report

> Miss Biagi was a 71-year-old single teacher with metastatic pancreatic cancer whose only support was her 68-year-old brother. Despite her symptoms of a reactive depression, Miss Biagi expressed a desire to die at home, and her physician referred her to the Home Care Program. With the initiation of pharmacological interventions of antidepressants and weekly supportive therapy at home by the nurse, Miss Biagi's emotional outlook improved. Her chief medical complaint was abdominal pain and severe bouts of nausea and vomiting. Miss Biagi's pain was initially controlled with oral morphine, but the progression of pain and increased severity of her nausea and vomiting led to the need for alternative routes of administration of analgesics. The desirability of using a continuous PCA pump was apparent to the home care team, but Miss Biagi had only limited funds and limited insurance coverage. The social worker was able to obtain insurance coverage and authorization for a PCA at home. The home care nurse was able to instruct Miss Biagi's brother in using the PCA. With continued instruction, he became proficient in monitoring and evaluating the need for additional rescue dosages and could even trouble-shoot the equipment when it malfunctioned. However, he was extremely fearful of giving Miss Biagi an overdose, despite the nurse's reassurance that the dosage was predetermined by the doctor. Despite continued reassurance, his own anxiety, feelings of inadequacy, and questioning the appropriateness of the PCA were continually disruptive. While discussing alternative routes of administration, Miss Biagi was readmitted to the hospital for a nerve block procedure to manage her pain more effectively. Once admitted, she and her brother were again instructed in using the PCA. When she was discharged home to her brother's house, both were completely comfortable and proficient with this technique, and she was able to be maintained pain free until her death.

Schachter observed that the level of physical symptoms is highly correlated with the level of physical exhaustion of the caregiver

(1992). Families often underestimate the physical aspects of home care, thinking only of the emotional upheavals and the anticipation of death. They do not consider and are not aware of the mountain of laundry—comprised of bedclothes and diapers—that must be washed daily. Few family caregivers are aware in advance of the amount of physical care required and the emotional fragility of the dying person. Schachter also noted that the feeling of "things being out of control" related to inadequate supports. Sleepless nights, hectic days, little support, and a feeling of being "alone with the problem" have a high correlation with the development of physical exhaustion in the caregiver. The following case illustrates caregiver fatigue.

Case Report

> Mr. and Mrs. Goldstein were a loving, elderly couple, married for eighteen years. He had limited interactions with his daughter from a previous marriage, and there were no family members living nearby. While on vacation Mr. Goldstein suffered a seizure and was diagnosed as having a glioblastoma. They returned home, and his wife assumed an active, primary role as caregiver. Despite surgical resection, external radiation treatments, and numerous courses of chemotherapy, the disease progressed. Home care management became increasingly difficult. Toward the end of her husband's life, Mrs. Goldstein wanted to keep him at home, knowing that in previous discussions he had expressed his desire to die there. Her ability to care for him would wax and wane, depending on her husband's physical and mental deterioration. Mr. Goldstein became forgetful and confused at times, with acute changes in mental status and episodes of delirium. Although Mrs. Goldstein had the finances and the ability to hire companions and home health aides to assist her with Mr. Goldstein, she insisted on doing everything herself. She felt the need to bathe and feed him herself. Mrs. Goldstein's fatigue increased as her husband's physical demands increased. Her health deteriorated as her arthritis and diabetes became exacerbated. Mrs. Goldstein was physically exhausted. She was unable to sleep at night, often waking up to change Mr. Goldstein, who was incontinent of both urine and stool. Days would go by without her leaving their apartment. She became depressed and described feeling like a prisoner in the home, yet feeling too guilty to relinquish any control.
>
> Once they were accepted into the Home Care Program, the primary nursing intervention centered on supporting Mrs. Goldstein and giving her "permission" to get help and spend time attending to her own needs. This was not an easy process, but over time a trusting relationship developed between the nurse and Mrs. Goldstein, making it easier for Mrs.

Goldstein to allow others to help her. Eventually she felt safe enough to lie down and nap during the day and even visit with neighbors.

The drain of the physical aspects of care are often rivaled by the psychological stresses. Jensen and Given (1991) noted that physical exhaustion is compounded by the anxiety and uncertainty about the timing of death and the way it may occur. Coupled with this is the strain for both the patient and the relative. The patient becomes humiliated by dependency, and the caregiver becomes overwhelmed by the many unfamiliar new roles and their demands. Roles, such as homemaker or breadwinner, that were the foundation of the family's structure may crumble, causing conflict and discord at the very time that closeness is most important. These roles are often taken over by other family members, who may or may not be prepared for them (Gonda and Ruark 1984). In addition, the patient may be unable to accept the loss of prior positions and roles. The burden of families trying to cope with impending death is increased. The following case illustrates difficulties with role reversals.

Case Report

> Mr. and Mrs. Campbell were a childless couple whose marriage centered around their professional careers as writers. Early in their marriage, Mrs. Campbell stepped back, encouraging her husband's career to flourish. Although she always worked as a free-lance writer, her primary focus was her husband's career as an international journalist. When Mr. Campbell was diagnosed with cancer of the tongue, they had no idea how profoundly his disease would affect their professional and private lives. Numerous head and neck surgeries left him disfigured and speechless. Because of issues related to changes in body image, Mr. Campbell became passive and was not willing or able to resume his former assertive role and responsibilities. Shortly after his difficult and painful death, Mrs. Campbell described her frustration after his surgery, when their roles were reversed. She tried not to "damage his autonomy" when she was forced to assume more of the decision making, yet she felt guilty about doing so. She described the remaining months as very stressful, and she was resentful at being forced to assume roles that she had given up earlier in their marriage.

An exacerbation of prior psychological problems, such as alcohol or substance abuse or personality problems that were successfully compensated for in the past, may also occur. Illness itself produces anxiety, depression, and often acute confusional states related to the disease process. It is particularly difficult for families to understand that paranoid delusions and hallucinations are organic in origin and are not based on reality, external events, or their care of the patient. Delirium occurred in 75 percent of dying patients studied by Massie, Holland, and Glass (1983). Hull (1989) also noted the high frequency of cognitive and memory problems that families do not expect or understand. It is imperative that the health care team not only try to control these symptoms but also patiently explain them to the family in words that they will understand.

The "silent sufferers" during the terminal illness of a person at home are often the children in the family. In a misguided effort, they are often excluded from discussions of the illness; they lack information shared by others about what is happening. The family secret of terminal illness is experienced by them as something terrible that they may have caused. They feel guilty, depressed, frightened, and isolated from the rest of family. They cannot share their worries with peers out of loyalty to the family. Withdrawal, anger, acting out, anxiety, and depression are common and often poorly identified or understood. The seeming lack of consideration for the ill person may lead to severe criticism of their "unloving" behavior. The health care team working in the home with children must be aware of the developmental level of each child and monitor their level of distress. Families must be instructed in the importance of including children in family discussions about the illness and its likely outcome. Death will be better handled if it is discussed and anticipated by the children as well.

Caregivers are at risk for significant psychological problems, and at times their distress level exceeds that of the patients (Given et al. 1993; Oberst et al. 1989). There is a strong interaction between the caregiver's coping and psychological state and that of the patient. Personal characteristics of the caregiver which show optimism and emotional maturity are associated with better outcomes for both patients and caregivers (Given et al. 1993). It is increasingly apparent that "helping the helper" programs have a payoff that is worth future study and investigation. The importance of respite care and community-developed programs that allow the caregiver to take a break from the burden of physical and psychological support cannot be overestimated.

Benefits and Liabilities of High-Tech Home Care

The benefits and liabilities of high-tech comfort care in the home for the patient and the family caregiver can be summarized to provide a clearer picture of the outcome of their use (table 6.1). First, for the patient, the benefits include being in a familiar environment, often characterized as the importance of being "in my own bed." At home, the patient interacts with the family more normally and informally, receiving support from family and friends, including sharing quiet activities while the daily patterns of living are maintained. Coordination and meticulous management of home care can maximize the patient's quality of life. The goal of controlling physical and psychiatric symptoms is a central benefit of care at home that is enhanced by the availability of home-based high technology.

The liabilities for the patient are fears of whether emergencies and severe symptoms will be able to be controlled, the absence of professional help "a bell's ring away" as it would be in the hospital, and fears that the family will become too tired or too stressed by financial problems to continue the care. The image of dependency on a "tether" is difficult for some patients who rely on external support of a physical function. Pfister describes the placement of percutaneous endoscopic jejunostomy (PEJ) or gastrostomy (PEG) tubes as a viable alternative to bypass the patient's digestive tract and provide adequate nutritional supplementation (chap. 4, this volume). The management of these tubes includes dressing changes and either bolus feedings (if tolerated) or an infusion of feedings using sensitive high-tech pumps that regulate the amount of formula infused over a

Table 6.1.
The benefits and liabilities of high-tech home care for terminal illness

Patient	Family
Benefits	
In familiar surroundings	Daily, informal contact
Interactions with family and friends	More control of decisions
More normal patterns of daily living	Sense of accomplishment with less guilt
High technology permits better control of symptoms	Anticipatory grieving; easier bereavement
Encourages autonomy	
Liabilities	
Greater fears about symptom control	Physical and emotional fatigue
Greater anxiety about emergencies and availability of professional help	Financial burden, present and future
	Insurance coverage is uncertain and varied
Concerns about family burden (financial, physical, emotional)	Disruption of home environment invaded by machines
Fears of abandonment; may lead to wishes for suicide or euthanasia	Loss of privacy
	Anxiety related to patients' treatment and maintenance of machinery

specific period of time. By slowing the delivery of the formula, patients are better able to tolerate and absorb these feedings and therefore experience fewer side effects (e.g., nausea, diarrhea, and abdominal cramps). Patients often complain of not only being tied to the machine but also of disturbing changes in their body image and loss of independence. This level of dependency has been most clearly seen in patients who describe a machine as an "umbilical cord." Families are instructed in the care of the machine, filling the feeding bag with formula, hanging the bag, and threading the tubing through the machine. The tubing is connected to the PEJ (or PEG), and the machine is turned on. For some families, this procedure is considered complicated and cumbersome.

"Psychological weaning" is a well-described phenomenon when patients are withdrawn from oxygen, protected germ-free environments, and respirators (Holland et al. 1977; Holland and Coles 1957). The guilt of using up resources (e.g., "my grandchild's college education") can lead to thoughts of suicide and sometimes for a request to "get it all over now." The public debate, as noted above, fuels the discussion now more than in the past, when the thoughts would have been unspoken. The following case exemplifies a loss of independence and being tethered to machines.

Case Report

> Dennis Kopelke was a 56-year-old married salesperson who had metastatic esophageal cancer. He had been treated in the past for anxiety and obsessive compulsive symptoms. His fifty-pound weight loss was the focus of his attention not only for its meaning about his illness but also for his devastation in acknowledging his changing body image. The impact of emaciation on his self-esteem and image was severe. He became isolated and withdrawn, refusing to see friends or leave his apartment. In an attempt to increase his nutrition and weight, he requested a PEJ, which was placed for supplemental tube feedings to increase his intake of calories. His wife agreed to the procedure in the hope of enhancing his self-esteem and appearance by the possibility of gaining weight. The PEJ was placed and they became proficient in giving the feedings. However, Mr. Kopelke's weight gain was minimal, and the feedings caused nausea, vomiting, and diarrhea. To reduce the nausea and vomiting, his physician changed from feeding by gravity to a pump to provide a more even flow of the feeding over an eighteen-hour period. This attempt was successful, but Mr. Kopelke became resentful of "being hooked up" and was fearful that something was going wrong. A battery-operated pump was suggested because he felt that the "tether" to an electrical plug was

intolerable. The feedings were also programed to begin in the evening, thus freeing up Mr. Kopelke during the day. A malfunction of the pump on two occasions led to increased anxiety related to the possibility of their inability to obtain professional help if needed. His wife became frustrated and overwhelmed with the care of his extensive physical and psychological problems; yet with the continued support and frequent home visits by the nurse, Mr. and Mrs. Kopelke felt supported. His condition deteriorated, and he died shortly afterward.

For the family, the advantages of home care are the ability to have unfettered daily contact and closeness without the intrusion of others. There is greater autonomy of patients and their families who are in control of decisions about care. The importance of such issues as directing that resuscitation not be carried out inadvertently by an emergency squad or that a death not be inappropriately made a medical examiner's case cannot be overstated. Planning by an alert, sensitive, and knowledgeable team with the caregiver can avoid those painful events. The chance to say last goodbyes and discuss issues of importance is much more likely to occur in a home setting and offers continued emotional support to the dying person. Additionally, the caregiver carries away from the experience the fact that "I did all that I could do," diminishing later regrets and guilt of abandonment. The period of anticipatory grieving is also enhanced with home care; the outcome of bereavement is more successfully resolved with a period of anticipation (Chochinov and Holland 1989).

The liabilities of home care for the family are several. First, the coverage for home care is spotty in most insurance policies, and the unreimbursed costs of high technology can run, extremely rapidly, into thousands and even hundreds of thousands of dollars. The tragedy is that even well-meaning families cannot manage for long without insurance coverage or independent resources. Medicare and Medicaid offer limited support for home care, and hospice coverage is limited in its scope as well (see chap. 5, this volume).

Case Report

> James Jefferson was a 43-year-old black unemployed Vietnam veteran with a long history of alcohol abuse. Born in West Virginia, he was living in a poverty-level, high-crime neighborhood with his partner of many years and their two children: a son, 11, and a 16-year-old daughter who was pregnant. Mr. Jefferson had mycosis fungoides, a form of non-Hodgkin lymphoma, which produced multiple skin lesions and ulcerations. His care was covered by Medicaid insurance. He had been ag-

gressively treated, without success, by high-dose methotrexate and bleo-mycin, radiation to localized areas, and finally total skin electron-beam radiation. He was admitted into the Home Care Program with diffuse scaling and plaquelike lesions, with widespread severe erythema and edema over most of his body. The lower extremities had peeling skin and sloughing, as well as ulcerations in the upper abdomen and left groin. To control the odor, these lesions required daily care with special chemical solutions and power sprays of sodium bicarbonate and normal saline. Mr. Jefferson's severe physical limitations caused him to be confined to his hospital bed and room. A trapeze and electric lift were used to get him out of bed into a wheelchair. His pain was managed with oral nar-cotics; he had portable oxygen by nasal cannula almost twenty-four hours a day.

Numerous family problems complicated Mr. Jefferson's home care. An older brother with a history of intravenous drug abuse and incarcera-tion lived in the same apartment building. It was feared that he would steal Mr. Jefferson's medications to sell on the street. Mr. Jefferson's partner had limited understanding of his illness and impending death. His care and treatment was problematic. The help of Mr. Jefferson's 72-year-old mother was elicited, and she visited almost daily to supervise her son's care. This was difficult, as she had severe arthritis and found it difficult to climb to the third floor where he lived. The elevator in the apartment house did not work. An infestation of cockroaches threatened the sterility of Mr. Jefferson's care at home.

The Psychiatry Service Home Care Program coordinated Mr. Jeffer-son's care with home health aides from a visiting nursing agency by tele-phone and with visits to the home accompanied by an escort for the protection of the nurse. Much time was spent working with his wife and educating her in the importance of not smoking near the oxygen, using sterile materials to clean his wounds, administering his medications ap-propriately, and handling the electric lift safely. Oxygen was the only equipment brought into the home that was covered by Medicaid. Any sophisticated technology could not have been considered because of cost. Daily telephone contact and weekly home visits by the home care nurse offered necessary emotional support to keep Mr. Jefferson at home in a safe environment. Surprisingly, over time, Mr. Jefferson's care was managed successfully at home. The psychological support of his mother and wife by the nurse made his home care possible.

Another liability is that high technology turns the bedroom into a hospital room, and the sense of invasion and intrusion is often great at times. Brown, Davies, and Martens (1990) stressed the importance of ensuring that the home environment does not become "eroded." They cited the problems of maintaining "normalcy" in the home and promoting the patient's independence while filling the home with supplies and equipment, thus making it a hospital environment. The following case illustrates a loss of privacy and difficulty maintaining normalcy at home.

Case Report

> Herbert Cheever was an active attorney who stated to his physician that he wished to commit suicide upon evidence of spread of his lung cancer to the throat. He was often in pain and experienced great difficulty in swallowing. He agreed to psychiatric consultation, and afterward stated that if symptoms were controlled, he would like to live for as long as he was comfortable and die at home. His wife welcomed his care at home but quickly found that they often viewed the twenty-four-hour private duty nurses, which they could afford, as an intrusion. An infusion pump was employed for analgesia, a PEG was given for feeding, and intravenous antibiotics were administered for an abdominal wound. A transfusion was given for weakness and lethargy. Mrs. Cheever expressed feeling excluded from her bedroom, which became a "mini-ICU." The sounds of repeated tracheostomy suctioning reached her in the other room, which she occupied, causing her much discomfort and distress. Mr. Cheever received aggressive palliative care with a good outcome for comfort; however, the loss of privacy and intimacy with her husband were negatives in an otherwise positive experience of terminal care.

Home health aides and nurses are needed supports, but at times they create tensions and conflict, making the family feel inadequate and displaced. The caregiver may feel isolated with the problem of few outside resources to call on. Access to the home care staff or a home care program is critical.

The emotional burden of day-to-day physical and psychological care is compounded by the daily thoughts about what the final event will be, how it will be handled, and what it will be like to live without the person. The caregiver has a sense of inadequacy and guilt because of not being skilled in the management of a medical emergency. This is coupled with the realization that the inevitable emergency associated with death will occur, and the family caregiver must manage it with as little discomfort to the patient as possible. This dual set of obligations constitutes a heavy burden.

Case Report

> Bill Deutsch was a 53-year-old gay interior decorator who had AIDS and Kaposi sarcoma. He had episodes of opportunistic infection that included *Pneumocystis carinii* pneumonia, toxoplasmosis with seizures, and

cytomegalovirus. He and his partner of twenty years managed with the support of a wide network of friends and family. Mr. Deutsch's lesions were disfiguring and painful and severely restricted his ability to ambulate. He insisted that he would not go to the hospital again, and the Home Care Program agreed to help him remain and die at home. Finances were limited, though some home care aides were available. His partner became exhausted with his care for pain control, which necessitated MS Contin (120 mg every six hours) and rescue doses of morphine sulfate (60 mg every hour). His lesions were irrigated with high-powered sprays twice a day to help relieve his pain. Over time, oral medications became impossible because of lethargy and his inability to swallow. Because of the absence of insurance coverage for parenteral routes by which to give medication, a nasogastric tube was placed not for nutrition but for medications that were crushed in a mortar and pestle. His partner's anxiety increased, fearing and anticipating an inability to give the medications needed to prevent seizures and control pain. Frequent supportive therapy and the initiation of anxiolytics was deemed helpful in supporting Mr. Deutsch's partner. Mr. Deutsch died at home in a coma with his loved ones surrounding him.

Conclusion

In our view, the benefits of home care clearly outweigh the liabilities. We believe that the liabilities can be minimized by addressing the family's needs in home care by discrete interventions. Health care policy must attend to the unmet needs of this growing aspect of care in our society. Families need (a) information and education about managing symptoms at home, best taught by a home care nurse; (b) communication with a medical care team who can present and discuss the medical issues in a language and manner that respects them as partners; (c) support and counseling, which must be built into medical health coverage; (d) increased coverage for home care, coupled with an examination of the high cost of home health agency services; and (e) more development of home care programs geared to the management of terminal illness at home. Programs that focus on the management of patients and their families during advanced stages of AIDS and cancer are needed and must be carefully evaluated for cost and efficacy.

REFERENCES

Bergen, A. 1992. Evaluating nursing care of the terminally ill in the community. *International Journal of Nursing Studies* 29:81–94.

Brown, P., Davies, B., and Martens, N. 1990. Families in supportive care.

Part II: Palliative care at home: A viable care setting. *Journal of Palliative Care.* 6:21–27.

Chochinov, H., and Holland, J. C. 1989. Bereavement and cancer. In J. C. Holland and J. H. Rowland, eds., *Handbook of Psycho-oncology,* pp. 612–31. New York: Oxford University Press.

Coyle, N. 1989. Continuity of care for the cancer patient with chronic pain. *Cancer* 63:2289–93.

Coyle, N., Loscalzo, M., and Bailey, L. 1990. Supportive home care for the advanced cancer patient and family. In J. C. Holland and J. H. Rowland, eds., *Handbook of Psycho-oncology,* pp. 598–606. New York: Oxford University Press.

Ferrell, B. R., Ferrell, B. A., Rhiner, M., and Grant, M. 1991. Family factors influencing cancer pain management. *Journal of Postgraduate Medicine* 67:564–69.

Given, C. W., Stommel, M., Given, B., Osuch, J., Kurtz, M. E., and Kurtz, J. C. 1993. The influence of cancer patients, symptoms and functional state on patient's depression and family caregivers' reaction and depression. *Health Psychology* 12:277–85.

Gonda, T. A., and Ruark J. E. 1984. *Dying Dignified.* Menlo Park, Calif.: Addison-Wesley.

Grobe, M. E., Ilstrup, D. M., and Ahmann, D. L. 1981. Skills needed by family members to maintain the care of an advanced cancer patient. *Cancer Nursing* 10:371–75.

Hileman, J. W., Lackey, N. R., and Hassanein, R. S. 1992. Identifying the needs of home caregivers of patients with cancer. *Oncology Nursing Forum* 19:771–77.

Holland, J. C., and Coles, M. R. 1957. Neuropsychiatric aspects of acute poliomyelitis. *The American Journal of Psychiatry* 114:54–63.

Holland, J. C., Rowland, J., and Plumb, M. 1977. Psychological aspects of anorexia in cancer patients. *Cancer Research* 37:2425–28.

Hull, M. M. 1989. Family needs and supportive nursing behaviors during terminal care: a review. *Oncology Nursing Forum* 16:787–92.

Jensen, S., and Given, B. A. 1991. Fatigue affecting family caregivers of cancer patients. *Cancer Nursing* 14:181–87.

Massie, M. J., Holland, J. C., and Glass, E. 1983. Delirium in terminally ill cancer patients. *American Journal of Psychiatry* 140:8–9.

Oberst, M. T., Thomas, S. E., Gass, K. A., and Ward, S. E. 1989. Caregiving demands and appraisal of stress among family caregivers. *Cancer Nursing* 12:209–15.

Sankar, A. 1991. *Dying at Home: A Family Guide for Caregiving.* Baltimore: Johns Hopkins University Press.

Schachter, S. 1992. Quality of life for families in the management of home care patients with advanced cancer. *Journal of Palliative Care* 8:61–66.

Siegel, K., Raveis, V. H., Houts, P., and Mor, V. 1991. Caregiver burden and unmet patient needs. *Cancer* 68:1131–40.

7. High-Tech Home Care for Elderly Persons

WHAT, WHY, AND HOW MUCH?

Lidia Pousada, M.D.

Geriatric Home Care: A Historical Perspective

We are currently in the midst of an unprecedented explosion of medical technology. Highly sophisticated respirators and oxygen-delivery devices provide assistance to, or completely support, a failing respiratory system. A broad spectrum of intravenous antibiotics aid the immune system in combating infection. A defective gastrointestinal system can be supported with tube feedings or replaced with parenteral nutrition. Dialysis machines take over the function of dying kidneys. A loss of normal urinary function is relieved by the use of catheters. Skin breakdown can be treated with air-fluidized beds. The neurological system can be modulated to provide relief from intractable pain with analgesics provided parenterally or via infusion pumps. Metabolic and endocrinologic derangements can be mitigated with the use of similar infusion pumps. Aberrant cardiac electrical activity can be treated with the use of implantable pacemakers and defibrillators. And the list goes on.

Over the past few decades, patients have crowded into tertiary care medical centers in a rush to benefit from "the latest." A technological hierarchy has evolved among medical centers, with the "best" centers competing avidly for funds and resources to support the most up-to-date biomedical equipment. Physicians are no longer seen as benevolent guardians; they have become the gatekeepers of this burgeoning technology. The quality of care, once experienced as the warmth and dedication of caregivers, is now gauged by the power and accuracy of machines.

Not surprisingly, this dehumanization of medical care has generated a significant backlash. The past few decades have seen a powerful movement on the part of the public toward increased patient autonomy, inclusion of patients and families in medical decision making, and recognition of patient rights, particularly with regard to the right to elect or eschew the use of medical technologies. In a somewhat ironic conclusion, this trend toward patient autonomy and a more "kindly," less institutional approach to medical care has coincided with the financial realities of prospective payment systems to create a "new" site for the deployment of this technology—the home.

Home care has become a catch phrase for a more caring approach to the sick and disabled. Who among us would wish to be institutionalized when we could be cared for in the familiarity of our own home? The World Institute on Disability summarized this sentiment in the recommendation that "no one should enter a nursing home or institution unless a finding has been made that they cannot live at home even with personal assistance" (Litvak, Zukas, and Heumann 1987). This issue is perhaps even more emotionally laden when one considers the impact of institutionalizing a parent or grandparent.

This ideological trend was markedly accelerated by the 1984 implementation of Medicare's prepayment system, with its emphasis on cost containment, and the creation of diagnosis-related groups (DRGs), which place a strict time limit on Medicare reimbursement to hospitals for given diagnoses (Champlin 1989). The conflict between giving optimal care and containing hospital costs has placed medical caregivers in an uncomfortable position. However, the pressure to discharge patients from the hospital "sicker and quicker" (Ferrel and Rubenstein 1991) has been mitigated by the consequent explosion in home care services. The result has been the creation of a large home care industry that revolves around the provision of personnel and equipment to continue in the home the same care initiated in the hospital.

Coincident with, and not entirely separate from, these developments in the field of medicine is one of the most dramatic trends in the history of mankind—the remarkable increase in average life expectancy that the advances of modern civilization have made possible. This "graying" of the population promises to have significant cultural, socioeconomic, and even anthropological impact well into the next millennium.

Curiously enough, up to the present this trend toward successful aging is largely accounted for not by medical advances but by industrialization and improvements in public health measures. However, it is increasingly clear that biomedical technology will play a key role in the further extension of life expectancy and the maintenance of the quality of life for elders.

Because of its relationship to disease burden, age is the most obvious factor relating to functional dependency and the need for home care assistance in the elderly population (Wieland, Ferrell, and Rubenstein 1991). It is reported that as many as 71 percent of home health agency clients are age 65 and over (Marion 1989). An estimated 2.7 million noninstitutionalized American elders suffer from a degree of disability sufficient to require assistance from another person in the home.

As more people survive into advanced age (85 years and older), disability and functional dependency increase. According to Manton and Soldo, the population 65 to 74 years old will grow by over 15 percent in the decades from 1980 to 2000 (Manton and Soldo 1987). In that same period, however, the segment of the population 85 years old and older has a projected 113 percent growth rate. In 1980, it was estimated that roughly 4.4 million American elders (18.2 percent of community-dwelling elders) suffered from some degree of functional limitation (Manton and Soldo 1987). In 1987, there were close to 5.6 million (19.7 percent) functionally impaired elders in the community. It is predicted that by the year 2000, the number of functionally impaired elderly in the community will increase to over 6.7 million, or 20.1 percent of the noninstitutionalized elderly (Manton and Soldo 1987). As more people live to very old age, there will be an increased need for home health care for chronically disabled, functionally impaired elders.

Thus it would appear that geriatric home care is here to stay, at least for the foreseeable future. The field is growing rapidly, both in the numbers served and in the intensity of care, with attendant demands for increased training of personnel and adaptation of current and future technologies to the unique needs of this sector of the population.

Specific Technologies Used in Geriatric Home Care

Among the technologies available for application to home care, several are prominent for their use in the care of elderly persons. Among these are the use of home emergency alarm systems, decubitus care with air-fluidized beds, the relief of urinary retention with catheterization of the urinary tract, nutritional supplementation via total parenteral nutrition and enteral feeding tubes, the administration of intravenous antibiotics, the use of home infusion pumps for patient-controlled analgesia (PCA), the treatment of kidney failure with chronic ambulatory peritoneal dialysis, and respiratory support via the use of home respirators and/or home oxygen therapy.

Home Emergency Alarms

The trend toward community care for disabled persons has led to a growth in the use of home emergency alarm systems. These systems are indicated for frail elders with a history of, or potential for, recurrent home emergencies such as falls. They are most useful in the socially isolated (e.g., the person who spends a significant portion of each day or night alone).

Inexpensive alarm systems such as cards placed in a window and systems of lights, bells, or buzzers have been used with minimal success. These all need to be activated from a single point or require patients to remain mobile and dexterous in an emergency. The response often depends on neighbors, which may impose excessive responsibility on them. Round-the-clock coverage is rarely possible, and the patient's vulnerability is advertised (Davies 1990).

Telephones can be used in emergency situations to summon assistance. Unfortunately, at least 6 percent of persons over 75 and 20 percent of those over 85 report difficulties using telephones. It has been reported that in 46 percent of accidents the victim cannot reach the telephone or dial.

Most emergency alarm systems are comprised of a home alarm unit, a triggering device, and a link to an emergency center. The emergency center is staffed around the clock with operators who have access to a computer database containing details about the resident and names and numbers of relatives or friends.

Triggering devices may be fixed (e.g., buttons or pull-cords on walls) or portable (e.g., pendant, clothes clip, wrist strap). Fixed triggers are problematic in that accidents often do not occur within convenient reach. Portable triggers are generally radio devices that activate the alarm unit from a variable distance. Some home units have a built-in loudspeaker and microphone that allows two-way speech between the resident and the emergency center. Some systems also function as smoke detectors and burglar alarms. Some require daily resetting by the resident and generate an alarm signal if not reset within a predetermined interval.

The advantages of these systems are obvious. The disadvantages include nonuse or incorrect use by residents, the creation of a false sense of security, and overuse or deliberate abuse. The demand for alarms has not come from residents, and alarm installation has escalated without any formal evidence of need or demand. The definition of the resident "at risk" remains nebulous. Nonetheless, the presence of alarms appears to be reassuring to patients and families; over half of interviewed residents stated that they would not like to be without the alarm (RICA 1986).

The alarm systems most widely used in the United States are not extremely expensive. Medic Alert, one of the most commonly used, requires a $75 installation fee and a $35 monthly connection fee. Other basic systems are comparable in price. Although these fees are not exorbitant, they are not covered by Medicare or third-party insurers and may represent a significant expense to the frail elder with multiple medical problems living on a fixed income.

Home emergency alarms represent an inexpensive use of simple technology to shore up an informal safety net for a frail community-dwelling elder. These devices increase security while supporting patient autonomy, a paradox that is rarely so easily addressed in geriatric practice. Moreover, they help keep elders out of expensive nursing homes and thus probably result in greater savings to society than have been documented to date.

Decubitus Care

Pressure sores (decubitus ulcers) are a recurrent problem for geriatric patients with chronic debilitating diseases. There is a sixfold increase in mortality when a pressure sore develops in an older patient; it is not clear whether this is because the development of pressure sores correlates with the presence of severe multisystemic disease or because pressure sores themselves cause an increase in mortality (Allman et al. 1986).

Geriatric patients with significant decubitus ulcers generally require the use of considerable health care resources, in terms of both caregiving personnel and medication/equipment (Melcher, Longe, and Gelbart 1988). Although the prevention and treatment of pressure sores was long considered a matter strictly of concern to nursing personnel, the rapid increase in the numbers of debilitated elders requiring aggressive medical intervention for the treatment of pressure sores has brought their prevention and care to the forefront of medical attention in recent years (Reule and Cooney 1981). Partly by design and partly by default, much of the financial burden of decubitus care has been borne by the Medicare and Medicaid programs (Strauss et al. 1991).

Although conventional wisdom teaches that pressure sores can be entirely prevented by nursing attention to frequent positioning, the increasing numbers of severely debilitated patients maintained by supportive therapies and the current financial realities of nursing and home attendant staffing call that teaching somewhat into question. In response to the decubitus "epidemic," an extensive array of skin care products have flooded the health care market. These products are generally expensive, but their costs are eclipsed by the financial impact of special bedding created for the prevention and treatment of pressure sores.

High-tech beds have been used in hospitals for decades, although financial considerations have often dictated a restriction of their use to burn patients and relatively young patients with acutely reversible disorders. Beds are essentially of two types: alternating-pressure air mattresses and air-fluidized beds. Alternating air mattresses consist of a series of baffles or compartments filled with air and connected to a pump that causes the compartments to fill and empty in a rhythmic manner. Air-fluidized beds contain beadlike ceramic spherules through which filtered air is circulated, thereby simulating the mechanics of "fluid" movement.

The principal rationale for using high-tech beds is to reduce capillary filling pressures in damaged tissues so as to permit or even promote healing. In addition, air-fluidized bed therapy is believed to eliminate shear and friction, reduce bacterial growth and pain, and increase comfort. The healing of advanced decubitus ulcers has been demonstrated to be significantly improved with the use of high-tech beds.

The disadvantages of these beds include possibilities for mechanical malfunction, the need for constant servicing, and the bulk and weight of the beds—significant limitations in home use. In addition, patients may develop dehydration and confusion related to sensory deprivation.

The greatest disadvantage, however, is cost. Whether they are used in an institution or home setting, these beds are extremely expensive. Rental runs between $50 and $200 per day, and outright purchase between $20,000 and $35,000. Randomized trials show no increase in cost between home and hospital. The use of these beds in the home care setting appears to result in a decrease in rehospitalizations and a greater capacity to adhere to DRG limits, which translates into some savings for hospitals but not for Medicare.

The use of high-tech beds for healing decubitus ulcers in elders raises several serious ethical issues. These beds are outstandingly effective when used after acute injuries or burns in younger patients.

Older patients who develop decubitus ulcers, however, are often immobilized, debilitated, and/or cognitively impaired. Thus, high-tech beds are a highly expensive treatment modality of dubious long-term efficacy when used in older patients with limited prognoses. The use of this technology on a chronic basis is currently viewed as debatable even in acute hospital settings. In the home, these beds truly represent the heavy artillery of the high-tech arsenal, and their cost, size, weight, and maintenance costs have caused them to be dubbed the "BMWs of decubitus care." Is this where we should be spending precious health care dollars? Many practitioners do not think so.

Urinary Tract Catheterization

Elderly patients not infrequently develop urinary retention due to either prostatic hypertrophy or urethral strictures in men, bladder atony (loss of normal muscle contraction) from central nervous system disease (e.g., stroke) or peripheral neuropathy (e.g., diabetes), or side effects of medication. As a result, a significant number of community-dwelling elders rely on the use of urinary tract catheterization to maintain normal urine flow.

Urinary catheters can be introduced at any point in the urological tract. The most common sites for placement are through the urethra into the bladder (Foley catheters) and through the anterior abdominal wall into the bladder (suprapubic catheters). Urethral catheters can be placed by patients, family members, or medical personnel and can be either indwelling or intermittent. Suprapubic catheters are placed surgically and are indwelling.

Urethral and suprapubic catheterizations are both relatively acceptable cosmetically. Indwelling catheter tubing is typically attached to a urine-collection bag that can be strapped to the leg and is thus not readily visible. Urethral catheterization can be uncomfortable, particularly when catheters require frequent changes.

Urethral catheters are relatively inexpensive but need regular changing. Suprapubic catheters are infrequently changed but must be monitored regularly by a urologist. The most common complication is urinary tract infection, which can be serious and frequently requires hospitalization in elderly persons.

Although the technology is not extremely expensive, urinary tract catheterization requires a certain amount of supervision by medical personnel. The costs of supervision are much lower for patients in the community than for those in institutions.

Urinary tract catheterization poses few ethical quandaries for most patients and practitioners. This technology is relatively nonin-vasive, is inexpensive, and requires little monitoring in the home set-ting. Since it resolves the management of urinary incontinence, this procedure often allows an elder to stay at home rather than require expensive nursing home care.

Nutritional Support

Elderly people often suffer from nutritional deficits, frequently as a result of neuromuscular deficits such as stroke or progressive demen-tia. Several approaches are available to maintain optimal nutrition in patients who are unable to be fed normally but have normal digestive capacity. The first is the placement of a nasogastric feeding tube, a flexible plastic tube passed through the nostril down the esophagus into the stomach. The advantages of nasogastric tube placement in-clude its temporary nature (the tube can be removed at any time) and its ease of placement. The disadvantages include chronic nasal irritation and discomfort as well as the cosmetic effect of having a tube in the middle of the face. In addition, a certain degree of gastro-esophageal reflux occurs, with an increased risk of aspiration pneu-monitis. Enteral supplement solutions frequently cause diarrhea, which can be uncomfortable for the patient and a management prob-lem for caretakers. Nasogastric tubes frequently become dislodged and need to be changed at regular intervals. Although the actual cost of a nasogastric tube is minimal, the use of the tube must be moni-tored by a home care nurse, who must periodically replace the tube.

Some of the disadvantages of nasogastric tube placement are ob-viated by the use of gastric feeding tubes. A variety of tubes are avail-able, but in the geriatric population the placement of percutaneous enteral gastrostomy (PEG) tubes has largely supplanted surgical tube placement because of their simplicity and cost-effectiveness, except in cases where anatomic considerations mandate a surgical approach. The primary advantage of a gastric feeding tube is its permanence. Although these tubes may need to be changed at infrequent intervals, they are well tolerated and rarely dislodged. An additional advantage is cosmetic. It is controversial whether gastric tubes have a lower inci-dence of gastroesophageal reflux and aspiration pneumonitis than nasogastric tubes.

Enteral feedings can be given either as bolus feedings (e.g., one can of supplement formula every eight hours) or as continuous infu-sions requiring a pump. There is evidence that patients tolerate con-tinuous feedings better than boluses; however, it is not clear that there is a lower risk of aspiration. Patients are generally positioned upright for a period of time after receiving a bolus feeding; this is not possible during continuous feedings. The use of an infusion pump increases cost.

Patients who cannot tolerate enteral alimentation can be given nutritional support intravenously. Total parenteral nutrition (TPN) is a means of providing calories, protein, vitamins, and minerals intravenously to maintain adequate nutrition in a patient at risk for compromise or to improve nutritional status in a nutritionally deficient patient. Home parenteral nutrition (HPN) is a relatively new application of this technology in geriatric patients (Vanderveen 1984). Until the early 1970s, patients with severe bowel dysfunction usually remained in the hospital until they died of septic or metabolic complications (Wilmore and Dudrick 1968). If they were discharged, their lack of nutritional support resulted in recurrent cachexia (wasting, malnutrition) and frequent readmission for dehydration and electrolyte imbalance. Since its introduction, this technology has received wide acceptance, and it is estimated that there are currently over 4000 patients on partial or complete HPN in the United States.

HPN is one of the most expensive new home therapies, usually costing $75,000 to $150,000 per patient year (Howard et al. 1991). To date, it has been used more frequently in younger patients than in the elderly. However, increasingly aggressive treatment of neoplastic disease in otherwise healthy elders suggests that the future will bring a greater use of this technology in the geriatric population.

The use of nutritional-support technology in elders has been the focus of raging controversy for some years. The spectrum of cases ranges from the healthy, active, physiologically "young" elder with limited or potentially treatable disease (e.g., cancer) to severely demented or comatose patients who have progressed to a permanent incapacity for oral nutrition. Very few physicians would advocate withholding nutritional support from the former type of patient. Unfortunately, problems commonly arise with the latter group.

Why do physicians use feeding tubes for elders with dementia? Severe dementia is, after all, known to be a progressive and ultimately terminal disorder. Commonly encountered reasons for the placement of feeding tubes in these patients include (a) a perception of food as being an "ordinary" rather than "extraordinary" measure, or of food and water (nutrition and hydration) as being "supportive care" rather than "heroic measures"; (b) the fact that the placement of a nasogastric tube is easy and minimally invasive; (c) a fear of litigation for having "starved" a patient to death if a tube is not placed;

and (d) an ethical mandate to save life and prevent death under all circumstances using whatever means are necessary and available.

It is likely that the controversy regarding standards of practice will continue when it comes to artificial nutrition via tubes. As a general statement, however, the "intermediate" practice of providing hydration without feeding should not be encouraged. This practice is often likened in lay terms to giving sips of water to an ailing patient who is too sick to eat. However, the reality is that intravenous hydration can provide enough water, sugar, and salt to ensure a slow death from starvation (usually months of recurrent infections and skin breakdown) rather than a relatively quick and painless death from dehydration (usually less than two weeks).

While there are few easy answers to the thorny issue of feeding severely cognitively impaired elders, the development of instruments and laws such as advance directives and the health care proxy has been helpful in this situation. Practitioners and institutions are much more likely to avoid reflex placement of feeding tubes if clear documentation of a patient's or proxy's wishes is made available. Perhaps equally helpful would be the dissemination of information to practitioners regarding the low rate of litigation in geriatric practice as well as information regarding litigation for inappropriate prolongation of a painful existence against patients' wishes.

Intravenous Antibiotic Therapy

Home intravenous infusion therapy is one of the most rapidly growing sectors of the home care market, with an estimated $2.2 billion spent in 1991 (Baxter 1989). The clinical use of home intravenous antibiotic therapy, first reported in 1974 (Rucker and Harrison 1974), has expanded enormously. This technology is of particular value to geriatrics because elderly patients' infections often require longer treatment than comparable disease in young persons. After the acute signs of infection have subsided, a long course of antibiotic therapy often requires only custodial care along with continued administration and monitoring of the drug. In addition, removing the older patient from the hospital environment reduces the risk of additional nosocomial infections. Thus, home antibiotic therapy is a rational alternative for elderly patients.

Not all patients, however, are candidates for home intravenous antibiotics. Clinical factors in patient selection include the stabilization of acute medical problems, sufficient patient independence and/or family support, the commitment of medical and nursing staff to close monitoring, the need for intravenous therapy for more than four days, adequate venous access, and the use of an antibiotic that can be safely administered in the home. Additional considerations include the capacity to train the patient and/or family members in the administration of medication, aseptic technique, dressing changes, the management of intravenous lines, and general troubleshooting. The patient must also have adequate insurance or financial resources available to cover the costs of therapy.

Virtually all classes of antibiotic have been used successfully in the home. Antibiotics are administered via the same types of intravenous access lines as TPN. However, it is important to note that home intravenous antibiotic therapy can be managed successfully only with a team approach, which includes a physician, visiting nurse, and home intravenous care company. The company often plays a critical role in the delivery of supplies, maintenance of venous access, facilitation of laboratory testing, management of minor complications, investigation of insurance coverage, and round-the-clock availability for troubleshooting (Bernstein 1991).

A new wrinkle in home antibiotic therapy has been the development of a computerized ambulatory infusion device (New et al. 1991). The obvious advantage of this system is a decrease in nursing time for dosage administration or for training the patient and family in dosing. The disadvantage is the risk of machine inaccuracy or malfunction. In addition, geriatric patients and their often equally aged relatives may experience difficulty comprehending or manipulating this technology.

The incidence of infectious complications on home intravenous antibiotic therapy has been reported to be as low as 2 percent (Graham et al. 1991), a rate that is as good as or better than that reported for in-hospital administration. On the average, the cost of home intravenous antibiotic therapy is one-half that of treating comparable patients in the hospital (Bernstein 1991). Unfortunately, Medicare does not cover this therapy at present, and it remains to be seen whether new legislation will alter this situation. There appears to be little ethical quandary regarding the provision of intravenous antibiotics to geriatric patients in the home versus the hospital. The primary concern is not the value of the technology but the availability of personal and supervisory support care. It would be unfortunate if frail elders were discharged home "sicker and quicker" with only an antibiotic-dispensing machine and a telephone number for back-up.

Pain Relief

Patient-controlled analgesia (PCA) is a relatively new but widely accepted approach to pain management in the acute care hospital, particularly for postoperative pain (White 1988). Home PCA permits select patients to deliver analgesia on the basis of their own perception of need. Most of patients receiving home PCA to date have been cancer patients with intractable pain (chap. 4, this volume), but this technology is increasingly being applied in patients with nonneoplastic disorders causing chronic severe pain.

It is notable that the concepts and practice of PCA are not new. The visible difference is the frequent use of a mechanized system to deliver analgesic medications. PCA is not limited to the use of a mechanical system; analgesics may be administered sublingually, via inhalation, rectally, subcutaneously, or orally (Bruera 1988). However, the frequent use of infusion pumps with indwelling catheters has led many to associate the term PCA with the use of a mechanical device operated by the patient to deliver pain medications. This has resulted in a somewhat slower growth in the use of PCA among elderly patients, in large part because of physicians' assumptions about the capacity of elderly patients and their families to manipulate complex mechanical devices.

Compared with other treatment modalities, PCA provides equivalent but no better relief of pain. However, it is generally preferred by patients, probably because it allows them to maintain a greater degree of control (McGrath et al. 1989). Patients for whom the use of PCA is relatively contraindicated include those with cognitive deficits, severe psychological disturbances, drug-seeking behavior, and insufficient educational or supervisory resources (Patt 1992).

The use of PCA in geriatric populations has not been quantified. However, it is expected that our increasingly interventional approach to the treatment of neoplastic disease in elderly people will result in significant numbers of elders using this technology. Estimates of cost-benefit are favorable, similar to the advantages of home antibiotic infusion.

The use of PCA in elders poses few ethical dilemmas. Even our society's chronic concern about analgesic addiction seems particularly groundless in a group of frail elders in pain whose remaining years of life are few and who are highly unlikely to take up a life of crime to support a narcotic addiction. Perhaps we should be more compelled by the opposite ethical dilemma—how can we continue to allow so many elders to suffer unnecessary pain at home when this technology could be mobilized to provide relief?

Continuous Ambulatory Peritoneal Dialysis

When a patient's kidney function declines to approximately 5 percent of normal or less, dialysis or transplantation is usually necessary. Approximately 250,000 patients (about half of them in the United States) maintain life without adequate renal function through the use of dialysis.

For several decades after its development, the use of dialysis was largely confined to university hospitals and was restricted to patients with potentially reversible acute renal failure. As techniques were developed that allowed prolonged dialysis, the patient population expanded. The passage of federal legislation in 1972 that mandated Medicare reimbursement for dialysis resulted in a rapid growth in the size of the population treated.

Home hemodialysis became available as a technique in 1964, but its complexity and potential dangers did not lead to wide acceptance, and the performance of hemodialysis at dialysis centers became the norm. Almost 40 percent of patients undergoing chronic hemodialysis were treated at home in 1972, but this proportion decreased to less than 10 percent in 1978 and has continued to decline further.

The technique of continuous ambulatory peritoneal dialysis (CAPD) was developed in 1976, and it rapidly became a popular alternative to hemodialysis. At present, roughly 30 percent of patients with newly diagnosed end-stage renal disease begin CAPD as their first renal replacement therapy (Maher and Maher 1989). Currently, more than 20,000 Americans with renal failure treat themselves with home dialysis.

The concept behind dialysis remains the same, regardless of the technique. The purpose of dialysis is to adjust abnormal plasma concentrations of certain solutes toward normal by diffusion across a semipermeable membrane. In extracorporeal hemodialysis, blood is brought externally through conduit tubing to a dialyzer, through which a rinsing solution flows. Access to the patient's blood is provided through a surgically created arteriovenous fistula, usually located in the forearm. The procedure lasts several hours and is typically repeated every two to four days. In peritoneal dialysis, the dialyzing fluid is introduced into the peritoneal cavity. After a period of time, during which the dialysis solution equilibrates with blood and accumulates toxicants, the fluid is drained and replaced. Access to the peritoneal cavity is through an implanted metal catheter, and bags of fluid are drained via gravity into and out of the peritoneal cavity. The procedure is continuous, with bags changed every four hours while the patient is awake.

A significant proportion of patients using CAPD are elderly, largely because patients who are old and frail have diminished cardiovascular reserve, or are severely diabetic are not good candidates for hemodialysis. Patient survival with CAPD averages roughly 65 percent after three years (Nolph, Lindblad, and Novak 1988). The bulk of the mortality occurs in the very young and the old; when only patients from age 15 to age 55 without coexisting diseases are considered, the annual survival with CAPD is greater than 95 percent (Maher and Maher 1989).

Significant advantages of CAPD include patient independence from machines and hospitals, a continuous and therefore more physiological dialysis process, no need for vascular access through the placement of a shunt or needlesticks, and better hemodynamic stability for patients with diminished cardiac reserve. In addition, diabetes can be better controlled, as insulin is added to the intraperitoneal fluid. Patients are often able to avoid the highly restrictive diet required during hemodialysis. Body homeostatic mechanisms appear better preserved, with more normal hormone levels and bone metabolism. The red cell count shows an average increase of 10 percent, because of higher levels of erythropoietin. In addition, the risk of contracting hepatitis is diminished. The overwhelming disadvantage of CAPD is the need to adhere strictly to a demanding schedule. Although patients can be trained in the procedure within two weeks and even blind and highly disabled patients have successfully participated, most patients require a great deal of family, nursing, and physician support to maintain the constant attention and energy required (Miller 1990).

Other complications of CAPD are peritonitis, catheter failure, abdominal hernias (which occur in 10 to 25 percent of patients) (Digenis et al. 1982), and massive pleural effusions. On the average, peritonitis occurs approximately once in every fourteen months of CAPD treatment (Maher and Maher 1989) and requires intraperitoneal treatment with antibiotics. However, patients can administer the intraperitoneal antibiotics themselves, and hospitalization is not usually required.

Financial analyses indicate that the annual cost of CAPD is roughly two-thirds to one-half that of hemodialysis (Prowant, Kappel, and Campbell 1986). Added costs related to the treatment of peritonitis appear comparable to the expense of the increased cardiovascular morbidity and shunt access complications seen in patients on hemodialysis.

Any discussion of dialysis in aged people must contain some consideration of the overall costs of both hemodialysis and CAPD. In some countries, dialysis is restricted or withheld strictly on the basis of advanced age. In the United States, rationing of health care resources has been regulated virtually only by the laws of supply and demand, as in the case of organ donations. Attempts at local rationing have resulted in "media-driven humanity" (Hafka 1985), in which individual appeals for resources are sponsored by the media. It is not clear whether the American tradition of "equal opportunity for all" can be withdrawn selectively from the arena of high-tech health care without a significant shift in the interpretation of our democratic tradition as well as a "desanctification" of health care technology.

Home Oxygen Use

The use of oxygen supplementation for respiratory insufficiency was reported as early as 1922 (Petty and Nett 1983). Oxygen supplied by compressed gas cylinders was used very sporadically at home in the late 1950s and early 1960s (Petty and Nett 1983). The development of a portable transfilling liquid oxygen system in the mid-1960s represented a turning point in outpatient oxygen therapy (Levine et al. 1987).

A variety of home oxygen systems have been developed. Stationary systems, such as oxygen concentrators or high-pressure cylinders, are preferable for patients who are essentially homebound. These individuals can still be ambulatory about the home, using fifty-foot tubing. Ambulatory patients, including those able to work, should have a portable system, which can be either a transfilling gaseous system or a liquid system. Most oxygen-delivery systems rely on the use of nasal cannulas, plastic tubing with two prongs to fit into the nostrils. These cannulas are relatively unobtrusive, but patients who breathe through the mouth may significantly dilute the oxygen mixture. Face masks that cover both nose and mouth are available; these provide more certain oxygen delivery but are generally cosmetically unacceptable. An interesting cosmetic adaptation is the use of nasal cannulas attached to specially constructed eyeglass frames, with the cannula approximating the nasolabial fold.

A recent development has been transtracheal oxygen administration, wherein a small polyethylene catheter is introduced via the front of the neck directly into the trachea (Christopher et al. 1987). Although catheter placement requires the use of a guidewire introducer as well as a metal chain for anchoring, it is an office procedure performed under local anesthesia. Patients are taught the techniques for cleaning and changing the catheter. The primary advantage of transtracheal catheter administration is that it provides much superior oxygenation to patients who require higher liter flow rates than are possible via nasal cannula (Christopher et al. 1986).

An additional benefit is the markedly improved cosmetic result, as the catheter can be entirely hidden by clothing. In addition, nasal congestion is relieved, and the senses of smell and taste (negatively affected by nasal oxygen) return to normal. Oxygen flow can often be decreased, thus improving the range of portable systems and offering potential cost benefits. The disadvantages of transtracheal oxygen administration include the theoretical potential of increased susceptibility to respiratory tract infection as well as local catheter-site infection. In addition, patients or caretakers must be trained in the cleaning and maintenance of a catheter.

The advantages of home oxygen use are considerable. Extensive evidence indicates that exercise is important therapy for chronic obstructive pulmonary disease (COPD); many patients can exercise only with the assistance of oxygen. Multicenter trials have clearly demonstrated that oxygen improves survival in selected patients with advanced COPD. Furthermore, the quality of life and brain function appear better when continuous ambulatory oxygen is employed (Heaton et al. 1983), and hospitalizations are reduced (NOTTG 1980).

The disadvantages are primarily financial. This is a costly technology (often $250 to $500 per month) with significant potential for overuse by physicians and patients. However, most experts in the field believe that the costs of long-term home oxygen are more than offset by reduced hospital costs (Petty 1990). It is possible that patients whose respiratory insufficiency is mild may become psychologically dependent on the use of this expensive technology; this issue is presumably avoided by current requirements for documenting a severe degree of hypoxemia.

Despite its cost, home oxygen therapy is widely viewed as appropriate for elders, in contradistinction to ventilator support. Some of this perception may stem from the relatively "low tech" quality of home oxygen delivery, and some may arise from its potential to decrease health care costs via decreased frequency of hospitalization and improved functional status. Perhaps most important, home oxygen use appears to relieve suffering and prolong useful life with few if any complications; thus, this technology is generally considered reasonable and appropriate for old people.

Ventilator Use

The most appropriate use of respiratory support via ventilator is for reversible conditions causing acute respiratory failure, such as exacerbations of asthma or COPD, pneumonia, adult respiratory distress syndrome, acute pulmonary edema due to congestive heart failure or myocardial ischemia, postoperative respiratory insufficiency, trauma, poisonings, and neurological emergencies. Unfortunately, it is not always possible to predict the reversibility of acute illness; in addition, patient and family wishes may supersede medical prognosis as an indication for the use of a ventilator. As a result, there are an estimated 11,000 long-term ventilator-dependent individuals in the United States at present (Bach et al. 1992). There are no current data on what percentage of this group is geriatric.

The benefits of the discharge of ventilator-dependent patients to the home setting include quality-of-life issues such as increased patient autonomy and reintegration into family life, decreased risk of resistant nosocomial infections, and cost-containment for hospitals and possibly for Medicare as well. However, disadvantages are not inconsiderable. Discharge planning is a complex process that must be coordinated via a team, which includes physician, nursing, dietary, social work, and rehabilitation staff as well as medical supply company personnel and family members. The caretaker burden for family members is considerable. Close and careful monitoring must continue in the outpatient setting, with a significant commitment from all the team members. Frequent rehospitalization is the rule, with pulmonary infections and caretaker stress as common causes.

What specific ethical issues are raised by the use of home ventilators in aged persons? Ventilators are life-support equipment. They prevent death rather than enhance the quality of life. In fact, it could be argued that life on a ventilator is generally of very low quality and characterized by much physical and psychological suffering (Snider 1984).

Most physicians would agree that the optimal use of ventilatory technology is to provide life support during an acute period of respiratory failure (e.g., an acute asthma attack or the early stages of a severe pneumonia). The provision of long-term respiratory support requires a thoughtful decision about the risks and benefits of therapy.

Long-term ventilatory support is much easier to justify in young persons, since the alternative—death by slow suffocation—seems so cruelly premature. Moreover, a young patient with isolated respiratory failure can marshal other forces to compensate for ventilatory dependence and can in fact live with a semblance of normalcy, as in the case of the famous young polio victim who married and fathered three children despite dependence on an iron lung.

However, the finite nature of life is a grim reality of human existence. We must all die, and we count ourselves lucky if we survive to die at an advanced age. What then is the practical purpose of delaying the inevitable by placing an 80-year-old patient on "long-term" ventilator support? Few elders with respiratory failure have no other concurrent diseases, thus their capacity to compensate is often minimal. The gain is at best limited, and the potential for complications is high. Moreover, the cost to society is not insignificant, and in an era of limited health care resources, the individual physician must be ever conscious of ethical allocation of expensive technology. It has been argued that we should not let young children suffer because of health care we give the elderly. Placed in that context, prolonged use of ventilators in elders could rationally be viewed as not only ineffective but also antisocial.

Summary

Geriatric home care is a rapidly expanding field because of the growing numbers of elders in our population, a societal movement away from institutional care, and the development of portable medical technologies. The trend toward home care suggests the development of "hospitals without walls," and the broader ramifications of this decentralization of health care remain to be seen.

The bulk of technologies currently in use in the home setting do not appear to be significantly more costly when used in the home than in an institutional setting. In fact, some of these technologies appear to be distinctly more cost-effective outside of the hospital. However, it is likely that entirely home-based technologies will evolve, and these may have serious financial and ethical implications for our society in the decades ahead.

A plethora of stances have been adopted with regard to our current policy of deploying high-tech health care for elderly persons. Most of these proposals center around the use of age as a threshold for rationing. However, there are several invalid assumptions hidden in most ageist health care reform plans. The first is that chronological age equals physiological age, which is flatly untrue. Health, well-being, and functional status do not correlate with years of life; individual variations are so great as to render this criterion useless from a scientific standpoint. Thus, choosing a single age at which to begin a limitation of medical therapies is erroneous when applied to individual cases.

A second common assumption is that high-tech medical support of old people is a burden that must be borne by younger workers. Although it is true that older workers often lack the muscular strength, coordination, endurance, and quick reflexes of the young, they can compensate for these losses with invaluable years of training and experience. As the average life expectancy has climbed dramatically in the last century, so has the functional status of the "young old" cohort between the ages of 65 and 80. Given our society's fixed focus on 65 as the age of retirement, it seems that few options have been explored for maintaining or enhancing the productivity of older workers.

Another common assumption is that elders are eager to use expensive technologies to extend life at all costs. As a practicing geriatrician, I have not found this to be the case. Most of my older patients are quite aware of and prepared for their own death. The current geriatric generation came of age in the early years of this century, when technophilia was not yet a standard American ideology. In fact, many elders express more fear than longing when they speak of doctors, machines, and modern medicine. In practice, I find it more common for middle-aged children to request high-tech interventions than for their elderly parents to do so. Perhaps this generation requires education regarding the inability of medical technology to confer immortality.

Given my experience in geriatric practice, Callahan's (1987) proposals in favor of encouraging elders to sacrifice access to technology in favor of future generations may very well be superfluous. Perhaps if practitioners adopted a more frank policy of discussing and documenting older patients' preferences, we would happily discover the unsuspected—namely, that the majority of elders request only the sparing use of medical technology and most choose quality of life over years of life. Until we as a society ask these questions of our old people, we cannot hope to shape a rational health care system for an increasingly geriatric society.

REFERENCES

Allman, R. M., Laprade, C. A., Noel, L. B., et al. 1986. Pressure sores among hospitalized patients. *Annals of Internal Medicine* 105:337–42.

Bach, J., Intintola, P., Alba, A. S., and Holland, I. E. 1992. The ventilator-assisted individual: Cost analysis of institutionalization versus rehabilitation and in-home management. *Chest* 101:260.

Baxter International. 1989. *Annual Report* p. 5.

Bernstein, L. H. 1991. An update on home intravenous antibiotic therapy. *Geriatrics* 46:47–54.

Bruera, E., Brenneis, C., Macmillan, K., et al. 1988. The use of the subcutaneous route for the administration of narcotics. *Cancer* 62:407–11.

Bunner, F. P., Wing, A. J., Dykes, S. R., et al. 1989. International review of renal replacement therapy: strategies and results. In J. F. Maher, ed., *Replacement of Renal Function by Dialysis*, 3d ed., pp. 697–719. Boston: Kluwer.

Callahan, D. 1987. *Setting Limits*. New York: Simon and Schuster.

Champlin, L. 1989. Home care goes "high-tech." *Geriatrics* 44:83–86.

Christopher, K. L., Spofford, B. T., Brannin, P. K., et al. 1986. Transtracheal oxygen therapy for refractory hypoxemia. *Journal of the American Medical Association* 256:484–97.

Christopher, K. L., Spofford, B. T., Petrun, M. D., et al. 1987. A program for transtracheal oxygen delivery. *Annals of Internal Medicine* 107:802–8.

Davies, K. N. 1990. Emergency alarms. *British Medical Journal* 300:1713–15.

Digenis, G. E., Khanach, R., Matthews, R., and Oreopoulos, D. G. 1982. Abdominal hernias in patients undergoing continuous ambulatory peritoneal dialysis. *Peritoneal Dialysis Bulletin* 2:115–17.

Feller, B. A. 1986. *Americans Needing Home Care: United States. Vital and Health Statistics*, series 10, no. 153. Data from the National Health Survey. DHHS publ. no. (PHS) 86–1581. Hyattsville, Md.: National Center for Health Statistics.

Ferrel, B. A., and Rubenstein, L. Z. 1991. Preface. *Clinics in Geriatric Medicine* 7:xiii.

Graham, D. R., Keldermans, M. M., Klemm, L. W., et al. 1991. Infectious complications among patients receiving home intravenous therapy with peripheral, central, or peripherally placed central venous catheters. *American Journal of Medicine* 91(suppl. 3B):95S-100S.

Heaton, R. K., Grant, I., McSweeney, A. J., et al. 1983. Psychologic effects of continuous and nocturnal oxygen therapy in hypoxemic chronic obstructive pulmonary disease. *Archives of Internal Medicine* 143:1941–47.

Howard, L., Heaphey, L., Fleming, C. R., et al. 1991. Four years of North American Registric home parenteral nutrition outcome data and their implications for patient management. *Journal of Parenteral and Enteral Nutrition* 15:384–93.

Levine, B. E., Bigelow, D. B., Hamstra, R. D., et al. 1987. The role of long-term continuous oxygen administration in patients with chronic airway obstruction with hypoxemia. *Annals of Internal Medicine* 66:639–50.

Litvak, S., Zukas, H., and Heumann, J. E. 1987. *Attending to America: Personal assistance for independent living. Executive summary of the national survey of attendant services programs in the United States*. Berkeley, Calif.: World Institute on Disability.

Maher, J. F., and Maher, A. T. 1989. Continuous ambulatory peritoneal dialysis. *American Family Physician* 40:187–92.

Manton, K. G., and Soldo, B. J. 1987. Dynamics of health changes in the oldest old: New perspectives and evidence. *Milbank Quarterly* 63:206.

Marion Laboratories. 1989. *Long-Term Care Digest; Home Health Care Edition*. Kansas City: Marion Laboratories.

McGrath, D., Thurston, N., Wright, D., et al. 1989. Comparison of one technique of patient-controlled postoperative analgesia with intramuscular meperidine. *Pain* 37:265–70.

Melcher, R. E., Longe, R. L., and Gelbart, A. O. 1988. Pressure sores in the elderly: A systematic approach to management. *Postgraduate Medicine* 83:299–308.

Miller, L. A. 1990. At-home help for the CAPD patient. *RN* August, pp. 77–80.

New, P.B., Swanson, G.F., Bulich, R.G., and Taplin, G.C. 1991. Ambulatory antibiotic infusion devices: Extending the spectrum of outpatient therapies. *American Journal of Medicine* 91:455–61.

Nocturnal Oxygen Therapy Trial Group (NOTTG). 1980. Continuous or nocturnal oxygen therapy in hypoxemia chronic obstructive lung disease. *Annals of Internal Medicine* 93:391–98.

Nolph, K. D., Lindblad, A. S., and Novak, J. W. 1988. Continuous ambulatory peritoneal dialysis. *New England Journal of Medicine* 318:1595–1600.

Patt, R. B. 1992. PCA: Prescribing analgesia for home management of severe pain. *Geriatrics* 47:69–84.

Petty, T.L. 1990. Home oxygen: A revolution in the care of advanced COPD. *Medical Clinics of America* 74:715–29.

Petty, T. L., and Nett, L. M. 1983. The history of long-term oxygen therapy. *Respiratory Care* 28:859–965.

Prowant, B., Kappel, D. F., and Campbell, A. 1986. A comparison of inpatient and outpatient Medicare allowable charges for continuous ambulatory peritoneal and center hemodialysis patients: A single-center study. *American Journal of Kidney Disease* 8:248–52.

Research Institute of Consumer Affairs (RICA). 1986. *Dispersed alarm systems: A guide for organizations installing systems*. London: Research Institute for Consumer Affairs.

Reule, J. B., and Cooney, T. G. 1981. The pressure sore: Pathophysiology and principles of management. *Annals of Internal Medicine* 94:661–66.

Rucker, R. U., and Harrison, G. M. 1974. Outpatient intravenous medication in the management of cystic fibrosis. *Pediatrics* 54:358–60.

Snider, G. I. 1989. Historical perspective on mechanical ventilation: From simple life support system to ethical dilemma. *American Review of Respiratory Disease* 140:S2-S7.

Strauss, M. J., Gong, J., Gary, B. D., et al. 1991. The cost of home air-fluidized therapy for pressure sores: A randomized controlled trial. *Journal of Family Practice* 33:52–59.

Vanderveen, T. W., and Niemiec, P. W. 1984. Parenteral nutrition. In E. T. Herfindal and J. L. Hirschman, eds., *Clinical Pharmacy and Therapeutics*, 3d ed., pp. 37–38. Baltimore: Williams & Wilkins.

White, P. F. 1988. Use of patient-controlled analgesia for management of acute pain. *Journal of the American Medical Association* 259:243–47.

Wieland, D., Ferrell, B. A., and Rubenstein, L. Z. 1991. Geriatric home health care: Conceptual and demographic considerations. *Clinics in Geriatric Medicine* 7:645–64.

Wilmore, D. W., and Dudrick, S. J. 1968. Growth and development of an infant receiving all nutrients exclusively by vein. *Journal of the American Medical Association* 203:860–64.

8. High-Tech Home Care for Elderly Persons

ISSUES AND RECOMMENDATIONS

Jeanie Kayser-Jones, R.N., Ph.D.

Today, it is argued that patients receiving home care have a higher quality of life than those who are cared for in institutional settings such as nursing homes. Patients who are treated at home have more control of their environment and daily routines, more privacy, and more contact with family and friends. Furthermore, it is believed that, when in their homes, elderly people are more oriented and retain better cognitive function (Wieland, Ferrell, and Rubenstein 1991).

In this chapter, I describe the experience of two terminally ill elderly people who were discharged from the hospital with the expectation that with supervisory visits from a home health care agency, they would be able to manage their complex treatment and therapy. Next, I discuss some of the major issues to be considered by health care providers when recommending high-tech home care for elderly persons. Last, I make recommendations to facilitate successful high-tech home care.

Data Collection

The data reported here were obtained using the anthropological field method over a four-month period (July to October 1992). Four strategies were used to obtain data: (*a*) participation observation in the acute care hospital and in patients' homes; (*b*) telephone interviews with nurses, patients' families, and vendors; (*c*) face-to-face informal interviews with acute hospital and home care staff and with elderly patients and their families; and (*d*) review of patients' hospital records. Physicians were not interviewed; I acknowledge that limitation.

I first interviewed liaison nurses in the acute care setting, the intermediaries between the nurses who provide the hands-on care in the acute care hospital and the home health care agency staff. From these nurses, I learned that while elderly patients were seldom discharged with high-tech equipment such as ventilators, many were sent home with oxygen, tube feedings, total parenteral nutrition (TPN), draining wounds, and decubitus ulcers. While some may not define these procedures as "high technology," for many elderly patients and their families they present a formidable challenge.

I next interviewed the director of nursing of the home care agency to learn about the agency's structure and philosophy and to obtain demographic data on the patients who use the agency. This hospital-based home care agency makes about 4,000 home visits per month; about 50 percent of their clients are 65 years of age and over. Three teams of registered nurses and home health aides provide home care within a large urban area. Each team comprises about sixteen registered nurses and three home health aides.

Returning to the acute care hospital, I began to visit patients who were soon to be discharged and then followed in the home by the home care agency. From among the patients visited, I selected two men, both with terminal cancer, who required high-tech home care.

Dr. Samuels

The liaison nurse in the hospital suggested that Dr. Samuels might be an interesting patient for me to follow. She added, however, that it might be difficult because "his wife is a physician, and she is a 'tippler.' " Furthermore the nurses had found her to be "somewhat of a nuisance" during her husband's hospitalization.

> Dr. Samuels was a 70-year-old man who had been a professor at a distinguished university; he retired eight years ago. After a persistent sore throat that did not respond to treatment with antibiotics, he was diagnosed as having squamous cell carcinoma, for which he received radiation therapy. At the end of this treatment, the tumor was no longer visible.
>
> About seven months later, a biopsy was done, and a recurrent squamous cell carcinoma was found. Dr. Samuels then had a left radical neck dissection followed by reconstructive surgery. He had been readmitted to the hospital several times for pneumonia and chemotherapy and now, because of air hunger, had been hospitalized to have a tracheostomy.

In discussing Dr. Samuels's case, the liaison nurse said, "This man is very intelligent. He is still very 'with it,' but his wife drinks, and he probably drinks too. You don't have a diagnosis like his without being a heavy drinker and smoker."

Dr. Samuels was discharged with a tracheostomy and a nasogastric feeding tube; I observed the interaction between two nurses as they discussed his home care. "The home care nurses are freaking out," one said. "They don't know how to do 'trach' care." I asked if the wife, a retired pediatric cardiologist, would be able to assist. "She's incompetent; I wouldn't trust her. She's an alcoholic," they replied.

On the day of discharge, the liaison nurse explained, apologetically, that she had not previously met Dr. Samuels. "I often do not meet the patients until the day they are being discharged. I am sorry but I just don't have the time."

I went to the room to meet Dr. Samuels and to ask if I might visit him in his home. The scene in the room was poignant. The patient's wife was sitting quietly in the corner. Her brother, visiting from out of state, and Dr. Samuels were at the bedside trying to organize the huge amount of equipment and supplies to be taken home. The supplies (e.g., dressings, gloves, and tracheostomy tubes) had been placed in a large plastic bag. Dr. Samuels was rummaging in the bag, attempting to find a tracheostomy set.

A nurse asked if he would like to change the tracheostomy tube before discharge; he did this competently. His wife was not invited to observe or participate; she remained quietly in the corner throughout the procedure.

I visited Dr. Samuels four days later in his comfortable home in a quiet middle-class neighborhood. When I arrived, he and his wife were waiting for the home care nurse, who was coming to assist in changing the tracheostomy tube.

Dr. Samuels changed the tracheostomy tube, both the inner and the outer cannulas, with some assistance from the nurse. By this time, the tumor had reappeared and was in a position that interfered with the insertion of the cannula. When he could not insert the cannula easily, he became anxious. The nurse quietly instructed him to hyperextend his neck and complimented him when the procedure was successfully completed.

A week later I called to arrange a visit to Dr. Samuels; his wife answered the telephone. "I called to see how you are getting along," I explained. "Me or my husband," she asked? She said that Dr. Samuels had gone back into the hospital for chemotherapy. Although his hospitalization had been scheduled, the admission procedure had not gone smoothly. "Listen to this," she said. "Neither of his doctors, the ear, nose, and throat (ENT) doctor nor the oncologist, bothered to tell the hospital admission staff that we would be coming." When they arrived at the hospital, one doctor was in surgery and the other in a conference, and nobody would interrupt either of them to get an order to admit Dr. Samuels. Thus, they had to wait for five hours before he was finally placed in a hospital room. "So yesterday was a rotten day," she explained. I asked how Dr. Samuels had tolerated the long wait. Did he become tired? How did he manage the tube feedings? "He was fatigued and depressed," she said. I inquired further about the depression. She replied, "He is so depressed that he curls up in a fetal position, puts his thumb in his mouth, and says, 'If everyone tells me I am going to die, then I will die.' "

"Does he know his prognosis," I asked? "Unfortunately, yes." Shouting multiple expletives, she angrily explained that the physician had told Dr. Samuels that he had only six months to live. "Pardon my French," she apologized, "but they told my husband his prognosis without first discussing it with me. I could have handled the situation if they had told me first. Let me begin at the beginning, but you'll have to give me a tenth of a second to get my act together." She was now crying.

At some length, she described an event that took place many years ago when she was practicing as a pediatric cardiologist. A patient of hers, an infant, had a serious congenital heart defect. The child was very ill, and the doctor did not want to operate. She went to the cardiac surgeon and asked him to operate, pleading that if he did not operate, the child would die. Although the child was a poor surgical risk, she persuaded the surgeon to operate, and the child lived to 21 years of age. "Some cardiac surgeons," she explained, "will operate only on patients who have a good chance of surviving. What I am stuck with now, in terms of my husband, is that I have this horrible suspicion that the doctor (the ENT) wants only those patients in his practice who will get well. If the oncologist doesn't want my husband on his record, then he, too, may write him off because he doesn't want a failure on his record."

The wife was also upset because she had overheard the doctor discussing her husband's case with the hospital residents: "He's 71, you know," the doctor told the residents. "I don't know what he meant by that," she said. "Did he mean he's 71, so nothing works; or he's 71, so the effects of the chemotherapy are too traumatic?" Whatever the doctor may have meant, Dr. Samuels's wife believed that age was a factor in determining the treatment plan. She remarked that they had not been treating her husband as aggressively now as they had said they would a year ago. "The time lapses between chemotherapy treatments are greater than originally projected," she insisted. "If they decide not to treat him aggressively, if they decide 'what the hell, he's too old, we will write him off,' then I am going to ask for a transfer to the Mayo Clinic, where he will be seen by people who *will* treat him more aggressively."

Sensing her anger and frustration, I asked, "And how are you?" "Mean, nasty, and belligerent. But I always win, no matter whom I have to browbeat. I haven't called a lawyer yet, but at the last minute I will." She named one of the most powerful lawyers in the area.

Mr. Bellagio

While the first case portrays the psychosocial problems that occurred during home care, the second case illustrates the serious complications that can occur when technology-dependent patients rely on home health care agencies to manage and monitor their care.

Mr. Bellagio, a 69-year-old Italian man, had been discharged from the hospital on total parenteral nutrition (TPN). Because of complications, however, he was readmitted to the hospital only a few days later. "It was a disaster," the nurse said, "and his wife was a basket case." Curious to learn why his home care had not gone well, I went to the hospital to talk with the nurses and to visit Mr. Bellagio and his wife.

Nine years earlier, Mr. Bellagio was diagnosed as having a malignant tumor of the bowel; the tumor was unresectable, and he received chemotherapy and radiation. One year later, he had a recurrent tumor and again received radiation therapy with resolution of the tumor. In 1990, a soft tissue mass was found. The tumor was unresectable; thus, part of the large bowel was removed, leaving Mr. Bellagio with a colostomy. He developed fluid in the abdomen, and two drains were placed, one in the pancreatic region and one in the left flank area.

In late 1992, Mr. Bellagio was again hospitalized; this time he was sent home on TPN, and arrangements were made for his care to be monitored by the home care agency. Complications soon occurred, however, and he was rehospitalized.

On the fifth day of hospitalization, the nurses on the unit and the liaison nurse became concerned. One nurse confided, "I'm getting the message that the docs want him out of here, and Mr. Bellagio is just a lump in the bed." I asked if he ever got out of bed. "No," she replied. "He is so depressed, and I am dealing with surgeons whom I never see."

The previous day a team meeting was held to discuss Mr. Bellagio's case, and a decision was made to have a psychiatric consultation as well as physical therapy and occupational therapy consultations. Interestingly, the physicians did not attend the team meeting; only the nurses and social workers participated. Later, the nurses decided not to get the psychiatric consult. "We don't want him to think that he's crazy," they explained.

In an attempt to reconstruct what happened at home during Mr. Bellagio's previous discharge, I spoke on the telephone with the home care nurse, a sensitive, caring young woman who was fond of and concerned about Mr. Bellagio and his family. She explained that apparently the TPN was too concentrated, and Mr. Bellagio had become dehydrated. When he was discharged, the doctor had ordered laboratory tests to be done only once a week. The nurse thought this was unsafe and that they should be done more frequently, but the doctor insisted that once a week was adequate. "I should have been more aggressive," she apologized.

The home care nurse said that during his previous admission, Mr. Bellagio refused to participate in his care, and he was adamant that his wife and daughter not do any of his care. "I think he wanted to protect his wife, or it may have been a cultural thing," she said. "I think he was a proud Italian guy who thought he should be taking care of his wife rather than her taking care of him."

When they got home and were suddenly faced with the complexity of his care, Mr. Bellagio and his family became very anxious. He had been discharged with TPN, an abdominal wound with two drains, and an old colostomy. "In retrospect, I think we expected too much in trying to teach him TPN along with wound care," she said. During the first two to three home care visits, she tried, with great difficulty, to teach Mr. Bellagio how to manage his care. Then it was the weekend, and when the nurse visited again on Monday, she could see that he had "really gone downhill."

When she arrived at the home, Mrs. Bellagio was very upset and speaking rapidly. The nurse said, "I wanted to say, 'just calm down, calm down,' but I soon realized why she was upset." She knows her husband, and she could see there was a serious problem.

Mrs. Bellagio said her husband was so tired he could not get out of bed, and he complained of severe thirst. The nurse called the doctor, who ordered laboratory tests. By the time the nurse received the test results in the afternoon, Mr. Bellagio had become gravely ill. "He was out of it," she said. She called the doctor again and reported that Mr. Bellagio's sodium level and hematocrit (a laboratory test that measures the percentage of red blood cells in the plasma) were elevated. The elevated sodium level and hematocrit indicated that Mr. Bellagio was severely dehydrated, and he was hospitalized immediately.

The nurse said she had learned a hard lesson. "Ideally," she explained, "the family should be told that if the patient is thirsty or dizzy, and if the urinary output is low, they need to call the doctor or the nurse." She had failed to do this. "I was focusing too much on the TPN line," she confessed, "and not enough on teaching them what to look for."

I asked if she knew Mr. Bellagio's prognosis. She replied that she had heard through the grapevine that it was not good. She also did not know if Mr. Bellagio and his wife knew his prognosis, but she said, "I would hazard a guess that they don't know because he is not being cared for by a medical doctor. A surgeon is caring for him, and they tend to put off telling people until the very last because they see it as a failure."

During the first home visit, the nurse had spent four hours with Mr. Bellagio and his wife. "I didn't mind spending that much time with him," she said, "But I guess as far as Medicare is concerned, it's not so good. And every time the story gets told by others, they exaggerate it more." The hospital gossip was that she had spent five hours on one home visit. "I'll bet she didn't do her six visits that day," the liaison nurse remarked.

When speaking with her supervisor at the home care agency, the supervisor emphasized, "We've got to put a stop to this. We're not a private nursing agency. I don't think he was an appropriate discharge." When the home care agency first accepted Mr. Bellagio, they did not know that he was going to have TPN. When they found that he was, they felt that they could not ethically refuse him, "But we do have to be concerned about the legal issues," the supervisor noted. As an administrator, she also considers the number of visits the nurses can make in a day for the home care agency to remain financially solvent. While there are no set rules, the nurses are expected to make five to six home visits daily. Interestingly, the home care agency receives a flat-rate reimbursement, whether the visit takes fifteen minutes or four hours. It is therefore to the agency's advantage to accept the less complicated cases. "Our role," she said, "is to teach people how to care for themselves and then to supervise that care, not to provide the hands-on care."

The Impact of High-Tech Home Care on Elderly Persons and Their Families: Issues for Consideration

While these cases differ in some respects, both portray the complexities of and problems encountered in providing high-tech home care to elderly people. They also illustrate the well-known fact that women (wives and daughters) bear the greatest burden of caring for family members in the home. Among the many issues to be considered by health care professionals when recommending high-tech home care for elderly persons are (a) the age and functional status of the care recipient and the caregiver; (b) the length of the caregiving experience and the patient's prognosis; and (c) the appropriateness of discharge from an acute care hospital to the home.

The Age and Functional Status of the Care Recipient and the Caregiver

In many cases, the care recipient and the caregiver are both elderly. Because many elderly people have physical and cognitive disabilities, the management of care increases in complexity and intensity as people grow older. A family caregiver may, for example, have to cope with urinary incontinence, cognitive impairment, and immobility along with procedures such as tube feedings, TPN, and wound care. Furthermore, a debilitated elderly person who is receiving nasogastric tube feedings is more at risk for skin and mucosal irritation and tissue breakdown than a younger person might be.

It is also important to recognize that the caregiver, who is often an elderly spouse, may have chronic conditions such as arthritis and congestive heart disease along with sensory loss (e.g., visual and hearing impairment), making the caregiving role even more difficult. The need to provide constant high-tech medical and personal care (e.g., bathing and feeding) along with the responsibility for meal preparation, financial matters, and other household duties may be exhausting and frustrating, resulting in fatigue, loss of appetite, and depression (Wilson 1990).

A 75-year-old person could, of course, be in better health than someone who is 55 years of age. Nevertheless, it is important to consider age, especially when the patient and the caregiver are very old (85 years of age or older). Among the very old, there is an increasing number of people whose elderly disabled children can no longer be depended on to assist with home care. Recently, I observed that a 78-year-old man had to institutionalize his 99-year-old mother (after a hip fracture); because of health problems, he was unable to care for her in the home.

Whereas some elderly caregivers may easily cope with machines and tubes, others, having lived in an era when such care was provided in hospitals, may be frightened and intimidated by equipment and procedures such as infusion pumps or tracheostomy care. When Dr. Samuels was being discharged, the hospital nurses remarked that the home care nurses were "freaking out" because they did not know how to do tracheostomy care. Yet, with minimal instruction, this 71-year-old man was expected to perform this procedure in the isolation of his home.

A reluctance to question or complain is often typical of elderly people. Many elderly people trust their physicians completely and are somewhat in awe of them. They may be reluctant to ask questions and to express their fears and concerns, and the doctors and nurses may fail to recognize that the family accepts the responsibility for providing high-tech home care for a loved one for emotional reasons, not because they are adept at or comfortable with providing the care.

The Length of the Caregiving Experience and the Patient's Prognosis

Whereas an elderly caregiver may be able to manage a short period of intensive care, providing care for months or years on end may be exhausting and unmanageable, resulting in neglect and in some cases abuse. It is estimated that elder abuse occurs in 3 percent of people over 65 years of age, mostly among those living at home (Pillemer and Finkelhor 1988). Wilson (1990) interviewed 188 elderly women who were caring for a disabled husband and found that 66 percent of them had been in the caregiver role for six to ten years. Eighty-five percent found the emotional and physical strain of caregiving exhausting and frustrating. They felt overwhelmed, isolated from family and friends, and concerned about financial problems, especially with respect to fear of costly institutionalization of their spouse.

An important consideration in high-tech home care is the patient's prognosis. With many frail elderly people, there is a continuous downhill trajectory. The burden of care increases over time, and the outcome is death. Conversely, if the prognosis is good, and the care recipient improves and is able to resume earlier roles, the burden of care decreases over time (O'Neill and Sorensen 1991).

Planning home care for a person who will recover is very different from planning care for a patient whose condition will progressively worsen. If the patient is terminally ill, as were Dr. Samuels and Mr. Bellagio, the elderly caregiver must cope not only with the complexities of high-tech home care but also with the imminent loss of a spouse. An important goal of home care for a terminally ill patient is to support the caregiver, who must deal with the reality of twenty-four-hour-a-day care, seven days a week, along with the emotional and psychological pain that accompanies the imminent loss of a loved one.

Dr. Samuels's care was further complicated by the fact that the physicians had not first discussed his prognosis with his wife; she resented this and was angry with them. Her relationship with the physicians was further eroded when she overheard them discussing her husband's care, making reference to the fact that he was 71 years old. She then believed that age was an important factor in determining Dr. Samuels's treatment plan, and it was her perception that they were not treating him as aggressively as originally planned. Thus, she had to cope with her husband's high-tech home care and his imminent death in a climate of mistrust.

The Appropriateness of Discharge

Today, in an attempt to control costs, hospitals are discharging patients "quicker and sicker." Because of the pressure to discharge patients as quickly as possible, there is great danger of sending people home too soon. "I don't think he was an appropriate discharge," the supervisor at the home care agency remarked when Mr. Bellagio was readmitted to the hospital in a critical condition. Yet, despite the serious problem that occurred when Mr. Bellagio was discharged with TPN, during his rehospitalization the nurses felt pressured to discharge him as quickly as possible. "I'm getting the message that the docs want him out of here," the liaison nurse confided.

An inappropriate discharge may be especially problematic for an elderly person who does not have the necessary resources to manage high-tech home care. In some cases, children live in distant cities and close friends may have died. Thus, there is little social support for the elderly caregiver.

Sometimes, as in the case of Mr. Bellagio, patients are discharged before they have been adequately instructed on how to manage a complex and potentially life-threatening therapy. Their care is complicated and may require several hours of nursing care a day. Yet some home care agencies are reluctant to accept such patients and do not want to increase their costs by accepting patients who need a considerable amount of "hands-on" care. This places the patient at risk and may result in a costly rehospitalization. When a problem occurs, it may make the caregiver feel that she has failed to provide competent care, and she may feel guilty, knowing her husband could have died because of her inability to recognize life-threatening symptoms. The patient, on the other hand, may also experience guilt, feeling that his care is too burdensome for his spouse. When complications occur, as they did for Mr. Bellagio, this becomes a stressful situation for the caregiver. The nurses described Mrs. Bellagio as a "basket case," and when the home care nurse arrived, Mrs. Bellagio was upset and anxious, knowing that her husband's condition was serious. An unsuccessful experience in providing high-tech home care resulting in rehospitalization will undoubtedly cause the caregiver to doubt her ability to succeed when her husband is again discharged, creating yet another stressful situation.

Recommendations

When an elderly person is discharged with high-tech home care, most of the attention is focused on the technical procedures, which, of course, are critically important. A thorough assessment of psychosociocultural factors and knowledge of past and current family dynamics and relationships, however, is also essential to the success of high-tech home care. Furthermore, adequate preparation before discharge and excellent communication among health care providers, patients, and their families is crucial.

Psychosocial Factors

Those planning the home care for Dr. Samuels ignored several important factors. It is remarkable that although Dr. Samuels's wife was a physician, she was not included in the discharge planning. The nursing staff, rather than taking advantage of her medical knowledge, labeled her a "tippler, an alcoholic, and incompetent." If she was not an alcoholic, she was labeled unfairly, and if alcoholism was a problem, it should have been dealt with professionally before the discharge. Rather than exploring this concern to determine if, in fact, a problem existed and if it would have adverse consequences for Dr. Samuels on discharge, the staff made derogatory statements about his wife.

Many studies have found that caregiving is a stressful experience (Abel 1990). Families with a history of psychosocial problems such as alcoholism or drug abuse cannot realistically be expected to provide complex home care. Caring for a dying husband is undoubtedly stressful and may exacerbate a drinking problem, adding further to the difficulty of providing safe high-tech home care.

Depression associated with physical illness occurs frequently among elderly people; however, it is not always recognized by health care providers (Finch, Ramsay, and Katona 1992), and in the cases presented above, it was overlooked. In a telephone conversation, Dr. Samuels's wife said he was so depressed that he "curls up in a fetal position, puts his thumb in his mouth, and says, 'If everyone tells me I am going to die, then I will die.' " Yet the physicians or nurses had not identified depression as a problem.

While a thorough medical history and physical are taken on every person who is hospitalized, health care professionals often have little knowledge of biographical facts and family relationships and dynamics. Yet ignorance of this information can have a profound effect on the quality of care and treatment outcome.

Wiener et al. (1979) noted that "an essential feature of medical-nursing work is that it is work on and with humans." Health professionals focus on assisting people during the course of an illness. When doing this, however, they must remember that patients and their families have a history and a life/biography that have some bearing on the work they do. Dr. Samuels's wife had learned from her professional experience as a pediatric cardiologist that doctors sometimes "write patients off." This knowledge, along with overhearing the doctor mention her husband's age, caused her to suspect that they were "writing off" her husband. "What I am stuck with," she said, "is that I have this horrible suspicion that the doctor wants only those patients in his practice who will get well." It was her perception that treatment was not as aggressive as previously planned. Perhaps the doctors had made the best decision regarding treatment. Unaware of her perceptions, however, they did not deal with her concerns; consequently, she became angry and mistrustful, adding further to her level of stress.

While the problems that Dr. Samuels and his wife experienced caused them psychological stress, Mr. Bellagio's care was compromised and his life endangered because of a lack of attention to cultural factors and family dynamics.

The family organization before an episode of illness has important implications for how families will manage that illness and high-tech home care (Harrison and Cole 1991). Mr. Bellagio and his wife had what Harrison and Cole described as a "complementary marital arrangement." In this type of marriage, the responsibilities for different aspects of family life are strictly allocated. There may be some overlap, but for the most part, the husband and wife each have certain duties and depend on their partner in other areas. When illness occurs, problems may arise because the partner who is ill can no longer take responsibility for certain roles. In this situation, the healthy family member experiences stress and anxiety, and the sick partner experiences guilt (Harrison and Cole 1991).

When Mr. Bellagio became ill, he was no longer able to be the strong husband and father figure. The nurses had observed that while in the hospital he was adamant that neither his wife nor his daughter do any of his care. "I think it was a cultural thing; he was a proud Italian guy," the home care nurse concluded. This issue was not explored, however. Furthermore, the physicians and nurses did not explain to him that it was unsafe to go home until he or his wife could manage his care.

Incredible as it may seem, Mr. Bellagio was discharged without knowing of the serious complications that could occur with TPN. Moreover, the home care nurse, intent on teaching him about the technical aspects of the TPN line, failed to discuss symptoms such as thirst, dizziness, and decreased urinary output, which indicate dehydration, a life-threatening complication. In this case, inattention to cultural factors may have accounted for the serious complications that occurred and the subsequent rehospitalization of Mr. Bellagio. In preparing families for discharge, in addition to teaching them the necessary skills, health care professionals must also address the issue of the healthy spouse being forced to take on new responsibilities in addition to her or his usual duties.

Communication

Nearly every family at some point will be faced with an illness that will require either a short or a prolonged period of home care. Many of the problems encountered by the two families discussed above could have been avoided or ameliorated if there had been better communication between the health care professionals, the patients, and their families.

Dr. Samuels

First, as mentioned above, the liaison nurse did not meet Dr. Samuels and his wife until the day of discharge. Thus, she did not have an opportunity to talk with them, establish rapport, and do an assessment to identify potential problems. She was unaware, for example, that the physicians had told Dr. Samuels his prognosis without first discussing it with his wife. Some may argue, of course, that it was appropriate for the physician to discuss the prognosis only with the patient. When the patient goes home, however, the family members will be the primary caregivers. Understanding their concerns and considering their wishes is, therefore, essential. Thus, while the wishes and needs of the patient are paramount, when information is given to the patient and decisions about care are being made, the family must also be included (Stephany 1992). If the nurses had talked with the wife, they might have learned that she wanted to be involved in deciding when and how to tell him of his prognosis. When she was excluded, understandably, she became angry.

Second, because of poor communication, a climate of mistrust developed between Dr. Samuels's wife and the physicians. Patient-family-physician communication is always important. When a family member is also a health care professional who has some "insider" knowledge of how health care decisions are made, other factors come into play. Because of her experience as a physician, Dr. Samuels's wife believed that the doctors wanted only those patients in their practice who would get well. She therefore believed that they had "written her husband off."

Further mistrust developed when she overheard the doctor comment on Dr. Samuels's age. The reference to his age led her to believe that they were not treating her husband as aggressively as previously planned. Perhaps the doctors had made the best possible decision regarding treatment, but because they had not discussed his prognosis and treatment plan with her, she felt angry, left out, and mistrustful.

Communication among the doctors, nurses, Dr. Samuels, and his wife might also have clarified the issue of alcoholism. Rather than exploring this concern to determine if, in fact, a problem existed and if it might have adverse consequences for Dr. Samuels upon discharge, derogatory statements were made. His wife was referred to as a "tippler, an alcoholic, and incompetent" without any factual evidence.

A major area of conflict among health care providers and patients and their families is in the sharing of important information (Harrison and Cole 1991). Arranging at least one meeting with patients, their families, and health care providers during which the patient's medical condition and home health care needs can be explained concurrently would facilitate communication and interpersonal relationships and improve the quality of high-tech home care (Dubler and Marcus 1994).

Mr. Bellagio

While communication problems contributed to the psychological stress that Dr. Samuels and his wife experienced, because of poor communication, Mr. Bellagio's care was compromised and his life was endangered. Today, many people on TPN are being cared for successfully in their homes. However, many complications, such as fluid and electrolyte abnormalities, glucose intolerance, catheter-related infections (e.g., septicemia), and thrombosis, can occur (Herfindal et al. 1992). These complications are serious and may be fatal. It is therefore imperative that patients and their families be well prepared before discharge and carefully monitored in the home.

Clearly, communication problems contributed to the fact that "a disaster occurred" when Mr. Bellagio was discharged on TPN. While in the hospital, he was adamant that his wife and daughter not do any of his care. Although the nurses had identified a problem, they did not try to learn why he would not let his family assist with his care. Furthermore, they did not explain that it was unsafe for him to go home until he or his wife could manage his care. It is incredible that Mr. Bellagio was discharged without being taught to recognize the serious complications that could occur with TPN.

Although it cannot be said definitively that a lack of communication between the home care nurse and the patient (failure to teach complications of TPN) occurred because home care nurses in this agency are expected to make five to six visits per day, the possibility that it may have influenced her judgment needs to be explored. The length of her four-hour visit was the subject of wide discussion. "I'll bet she didn't make her six visits that day," a liaison nurse remarked. And her supervisor said, "We've got to put a stop to this." If the home care nurse had discussed with her supervisor the need for a longer home visit, could the problem have been avoided?

In the United States, only about 10 percent of physicians make regular home visits. House calls constitute less than 1 percent of medical practice activity (Keenan and Hepburn 1991). Since many physicians do not make home visits, it is imperative that physicians, nurses, social workers, dietitians, and all those involved thoroughly discuss high-tech home care with patients and their families before discharge, to ensure successful home care. In the care of elderly people, because of multiple pathologies and functional disabilities, an interdisciplinary team approach using everyone's capabilities to the fullest will ensure the highest quality of care. Excellent communication among all concerned is critical.

Conclusion

The cases presented here illustrate the issues that health care providers need to consider when caring for patients and their families who are involved in high-tech home care. They also illustrate the tremendous need for improved communication and collaboration among health care providers, patients, and their families. Improved communication will facilitate decision making, improve the quality of care, create a climate of trust among all parties, increase satisfaction with care, decrease stress and anxiety for everyone, and in some cases decrease the cost of care by preventing rehospitalization.

Inevitably, there will be continued growth in the home care sector. It is somewhat frightening to see enormous responsibility for care being placed on elderly patients and their families. Today, we expect patients and their families to learn in a few brief lessons complex skills that it has taken professionals many years to acquire. Home care has many advantages (Collopy, Dubler, and Zuckerman 1990)—for example, it protects some people from being institutionalized, a fate many Americans fear—but we must recognize that even with adequate resources, home care places an enormous responsibility and burden on elderly patients and their families. Further research is needed to identify and analyze the impact of high-tech home care on elderly people and their families and to assess the quality of care being provided by home health care agencies.

REFERENCES

Abel, E. K. 1990. Informal care for the disabled elderly: A critique of recent literature. *Research on Aging and Health* 12:139–57.

Collopy, B., Dubler, N., and Zuckerman, C. 1990. The ethics of home care: Autonomy and accommodation. *Hastings Center Report* 20:1–16.

Dubler, N., and Marcus, L. J. 1994. *Mediating Bioethical Disputes: A Practical Guide*, pp. 23. New York: United Hospital Fund of New York.

Finch, E., Ramsay, R., and Katona, C. 1992. Depression and physical illness in the elderly. *Clinics in Geriatric Medicine* 8:275–87.

Harrison, D. S., and Cole, K. D. 1991. Family dynamics and caregiver burden in home health care. *Clinics in Geriatric Medicine* 7:817–29.

Herfindal, E. T., Bernstein R., Wong, A. F., Hogue, V. W., and Darbinian, J. A. 1992. Complications of home parenteral nutrition. *Clinical Pharmacy* 11: 543–48.

Keenan, J. M. and Hepburn, K. W. 1991. The role of physicians in home health care. *Clinics in Geriatric Medicine* 7: 665–75.

O'Neill, C., and Sorensen, E. S. 1991. Home care of the elderly: A family perspective. *Advances in Nursing Science* 13:28–37.

Pillemer, K., and Finkelhor, D. 1988. The prevalence of elder abuse: A random sample survey. *Gerontologist* 28:51–57.

Stephany, T. M. 1992. Home care for the terminally ill. *California Nurse*, June, 6–7.

Wieland, D., Ferrell, B. A., and Rubenstein, L. Z. 1991. Geriatric home health care: Conceptual and demographic considerations. *Geriatric Home Care* 7:645–64.

Wiener, C., Strauss, A., Fagerhaugh, S., and Suczek, B. 1979. Trajectories, biographies and the evolving medical scene. *Sociology and Health & Illness: A Journal of Medical Sociology* 1:261–83.

Wilson, V. 1990. The consequences of elderly wives caring for disabled husbands: Implications for practice. *Social Work* 35:417–21.

II. Philosophical and Policy Perspectives on High-Tech Home Care

9. Moral Obligation or Moral Support for High-Tech Home Care?

Nel Noddings, Ph.D.

As our technical capacity has grown in medicine, the costs of medical care have grown enormously. Costs—especially those for the care of severely handicapped, chronically ill, and terminally ill persons— have grown so large that they pose a threat to a host of other goods sought by our society. In such a setting, it is not surprising that policymakers and other thinkers have begun to ask who should be responsible for various forms of care. It would once have been unthinkable to ask whether parents were responsible for their children's health care and almost unthinkable to ask whether adult children should be responsible for the care of their elderly parents. Today such questions are being pressed (Callahan 1985). They are often posed as questions of moral obligation and the limits of moral obligation.

In this chapter, I approach the problem differently. First, I argue that we might do better to emphasize moral support rather than moral obligation. This move focuses our attention on the whole network of care and suffering and not on individual moral agents. Second, I take a close look at this network and develop an analysis that takes into account not only the sufferings of a victim or patient and of the whole society but also those of particular others in the network. My analysis is, at least in part, feminist inasmuch as it recognizes that proposed programs of home care often implicitly endorse the continued exploitation of women. But, more important, it is feminist in its emphasis on care and relation over abstract ethical principle and individual moral agency.

The chapter closes with a recommendation that we adopt a response-to-need orientation in health care. On first glance, such an orientation seems highly idealistic, and in one sense it is. Taking such a recommendation seriously necessitates a thorough analysis and re-working not just of health care policies but of public policies in hous-ing, child care, and education as well. It also requires an analytical emphasis on reducing the costs of services and supporting the least expensive equipment and personnel rather than on reducing or cut-ting services. But, in another sense, the recommendation is ultimately practical; such analyses are badly needed before important decisions are made. Further, the recommendation itself conforms to widely rec-ognized human insights and, especially, to some that have arisen in female experience.

Natural Caring and Moral Support

When policymakers begin an analysis of health care with a discussion of moral obligation, they are usually seeking firm rules to guide policy and sometimes are even anticipating laws to enforce certain behav-iors. For example, having decided that under most conditions, fathers have a moral obligation to support their minor children, we feel justi-fied in encoding the obligation in law and enforcing it. Correspond-ingly, if we were to decide that adult children have a moral obligation to care for their elderly parents, we might well describe this obligation legally and create the machinery to enforce it.

Such a strategy is likely to be ineffective in two important ways: it may well be more expensive than giving direct help to those willing to provide care, and, worse, it may contribute to the deterioration, rather than enhancement, of natural caring. Consider the case of Mr. Clark, an elderly man in need of nursing care. He is the father of seven living children, but only one will have anything to do with him. Social workers and strangers describe him as a sweet and funny old man. But his children remember him as a cruel father who de-serted their mother and abused them regularly. Now, of course, no one initially involved in the case would know about Mr. Clark's unsa-vory past because the eldest daughter, who is willing to assume some obligation, will not divulge this information. It could emerge only through an investigation, and investigations cost money.

Let's suppose we had a law that said all of the children had to contribute to their father's care. The investigators would first have to locate the children. One daughter is reasonably well off and agrees, reluctantly, to contribute the minimum required. Another is a widow in public housing and can give nothing. A third, with a long history of mental illness, refuses to contribute. With an unstable employment record and a habit of moving about constantly, she will lead investigators on a merry search, for little, if any, return. All three sons have deserted their own families and will be hard to locate. Should they be pursued? By now, the social workers know that the "sweet old man" was a holy terror and that his children have good reason to hate him, but the law does not discriminate between good and bad elderly fathers.

In actual life, without a law based on moral obligation, Mr. Clark's oldest daughter turned to her husband, two adult daughters, and a son-in-law, who were willing to help in finding a nursing home, providing transportation, making visits, arranging for laundry, and the like. This is the network of care that needs recognition and support. The pursuit of unwilling contributors may, on occasion, yield a quick and positive financial balance, but it will also increase an already bloated bureaucracy that is itself enormously costly, and it may very well erode the network of care further. Under such policies of enforcement, even willing contributors begin to explore their own rights and how little they must give to meet the minimum legal requirement.

A better way to begin is to assume that most people who have experienced care themselves want to care for their loved ones. The task of an enlightened society is to help them do so, and this help falls naturally into two large categories: (*a*) devising social and educational policies likely to produce adults who have themselves been cared for and, therefore, are prepared and willing to care, and (*b*) providing the kind of support needed by particular caregivers in particular situations. The first is far too large a topic to consider here, but I need to say a little about its theoretical underpinnings to make my analysis of the second plausible.

An ethic of care (Noddings 1984) inverts Kantian priorities. Kant insisted that ethical acts are those done out of duty (defined logically and derived from logical principles) and that acts performed out of personal love have no moral status. Hence, duty has a higher priority than love or compassionate inclination. In an ethic of care, however, caring out of love or inclination—what we might call natural caring—has a higher priority than ethical caring, and ethical caring is invoked primarily to create, restore, or enhance the preferred state. Even here, the senses of obligation in Kantian ethics and in an ethic of care are very different. Whereas duty is defined in terms of rules logically derived from principles in Kantian ethics, the duties of ethical caring arise out of memories of caring and being cared for and the value placed on caring relations. More rarely, ethical caring is constructed in some individuals through imagination and vicarious experience. In this case, too, a high value is placed on the caring relations dreamed of and longed for.

Ethical caring, caring that has to be summoned—by obedience to duty and principle in Kantian ethics, by reminders of an ideal self in caring—always lacks something. In personal relations, it often lacks warmth, because carers are drawing on something to replace their usual inclination to care. Astute recipients of care can often detect a subtle difference, and this difference is a main complaint directed at public caregiving (Waerness 1984). In interactions with strangers or in diplomatic and political relations, ethical caring is often employed because we lack information; we have not had time to develop caring relations. In such situations, we respond to strangers by rule or as we think they might want us to, if they are like other people we know. In some systems of ethics, we even count detachment as a significant virtue and rely on abstract rules of justice or the optimization of happiness—defined, of course, in terms familiar to *us*. However, in ordinary life, detachment is rarely considered a virtue, and agents and recipients feel the lack and instability in ethical caring; they long for eye contact, conversation, and opportunities to see and hear for themselves what others are going through. They believe, with Simone Weil (1977), that the question, "What are you going through?" put to another explicitly or implicitly by one's attentive presence, is essential to moral life. Asking this question requires, as Weil pointed out, attention directed at the recipient of our care. In ethical caring, as contrasted with natural caring, part of our attention is necessarily on ourselves because we have to ask what our best self would do in this situation or what we might do to restore natural caring. Ethical caring is clearly important, but it serves natural caring; it cannot supplant it.

Even relations usually governed by natural caring—family relations, friendships—require the occasional use of ethical caring. When we are tired or out of sorts, when our spouses or children behave obnoxiously, when conditions overwhelm us, we have to draw on the resources associated with ethical caring. In Kantian ethics, we turn to an analysis of principles and duty; in caring, we turn to our memories of caring and being cared for—to a vision of our best selves. We remind ourselves how we would respond if we were feeling better and the other were, perhaps, behaving better. The enterprise is risky. Because it requires control and effort, we are conscious of our own goodness, and we may lose patience in a fit of self-righteousness. Or, we may succeed all too well and contribute simultaneously to our own exploitation and the diminution of the other's moral self. Both phenomena are revealed in powerful case studies of caregiving now available to us (Abel 1991; Gubrium 1991; McNulty and Dann 1985; Silverstone and Hyman 1976; Sommers and Shields 1987). The fear of such unwanted results complicates relations at every level of human interaction.

When we recognize that natural caring is both the means and the end of ethical caring—that is, that the capacity for ethical care develops out of natural caring and the purpose of ethical care is to restore natural care—we are ready to explore a different approach to moral life and to public policy. Instead of establishing and trying to enforce rules based on a notion of minimal moral obligation, we ask how we can encourage the highest possible level of natural caring. Instead of forcing people to do their fair share, even if reluctantly, we ask what the public can do to make it more likely that people will want to care for others. This approach has many implications for education (Noddings 1992) and for public policy generally. For present purposes, it suggests a thorough analysis of capacities and sufferings throughout the network of care.

Suffering and the Capacity to Care

In the following analysis, I do not mean to suggest that every potential caregiver must be evaluated meticulously in each and every category. Rather, professionals in medicine and social work should be aware of the questions and issues. They should ask, implicitly at least, "What are you going through?" and the question should be put explicitly when there is evidence to suggest stress and suffering. Also, booklets for caregivers could be written covering all of these matters, and policies could be drawn with them in mind. The issues are organized around four major questions: (*a*) What do these people mean to each other? (*b*) What are the caregivers' capacities and projects? (*c*) What are the positive and negative features of the home's facilities, and what do these mean to the people who live there? and (*d*) Who is suffering?

What Do These People Mean to Each Other?

Mrs. Traub describes how much easier it was to care for one of her children through a serious illness and long recovery confined to bed than to provide ordinary care and companionship for her elderly mother, who now lives with Mr. and Mrs. Traub. Mrs. Traub loved her little daughter dearly, and, with proper care, complete recovery was predicted; this positive prognosis was, clearly, significant in relieving the burdens associated with home care. As Mrs. Traub describes it, her daughter's "sick room" was a place filled with learning, fun, and companionship. The other children loved spending time there, and Mrs. Traub found the caregiving chores easy to carry out. The child recovered, and hope had always been a part of what sustained and strengthened the family. But the bond between the child, Wendy, and her mother was paramount. The two loved each other and delighted in each other's company. That love has continued into Wendy's adulthood.

In contrast, Mrs. Traub's mother—"Grandma"—does not have the vibrant intelligence and sunny disposition of Wendy. She is physically healthy but has lost most of her mental capacity. She asks the same questions over and over and becomes angry when people point this out to her. She often complains that no one told her about upcoming events, even though the events have been discussed many times. Other family members find her difficult, and visits are becoming fewer and fewer. She needs some help with physical care but will not acknowledge the need. Getting her to bathe or shower is a constant hassle. But, for Mrs. Traub, it is worse than a hassle. She feels guilty because she dislikes touching her mother. Something in a smothering past makes her pull away. In contrast, she enjoyed lifting, holding, bathing, and caressing her little daughter. Her daughter was and remains special in her life. She has to draw on ethical caring to provide for her mother, and even with effort, she often feels unsuccessful and guilty.

When people are called on to become caregivers—whether or not that care requires handling technology—it is important to know what caregivers and cared-fors mean to each other and to assess the strength of relations throughout the web of care. We cannot decide on the basis of formal relations what one person owes another. We ordinarily think of parents having an almost total obligation to care for their children, but one can imagine a mother less than eager to care for a semicomatose teenager who overdosed on drugs after repeated efforts to "keep him clean." One can also imagine with some sympathy the resentment a parent may feel toward a child who claims so much attention that other children in the family feel unloved or neglected. Further, the other children are fun to be with, and the parents know that they themselves—as well as the children—are missing that fun, and they feel guilty.

The question, "What do these people mean to each other?" is especially important when the patient is an adult. An elderly parent—like Mr. Clark—may have been a nasty parent, and one can hardly expect children to respond lovingly to his present needs. Indeed, if the question of what they mean to each other is answered in terms of fear, anger, resentment, disgust, or contempt, home care should probably be discouraged.

Ideally, collective financial responsibility would make it possible for families and professionals to make the best practical choice without concern about individual financial burdens. The responsibility for financial management would also fall into the public domain, and professionals would be asked to manage public monies and services as carefully as most of us do our own private funds. Serious efforts would be made to keep all forms of care as financially effective as possible, but the choice of which form should be available to a given family should be made on human grounds, not financial ones. Such public provision might look very like the flexible care plans and "benefit menus" now proposed by various group insurance programs. When we know what people mean to each other and that home care is at least a psychologically feasible possibility (Kohrman 1991), we are ready to ask the next round of questions.

What Are the Caregivers' Capacities and Projects?

Most writers on high-tech home care consider the training required for caregivers (Crystal et al. 1987; OTA 1987). Providing for the patient's emotional needs is also sometimes included in the training or selection of caregivers. But beyond a brief recognition that an appropriate attitude and adequate technical training are required, it is often assumed that almost anyone can be prepared to administer high-tech home care. Much attention is given to the quality of training; not much attention is given to the caregiver's emotional needs.

From a feminist perspective, the most deplorable assumption made by both professionals and laypersons is that caregiving is the natural domain of women and that the closest female relation has the duty to provide care (Abel 1991). Traditionally, the only acceptable excuse a woman has been able to offer is competing duties to care. Thus, a woman with several small children might be able to suggest, without guilt or shame, that her unmarried sister accept the duty to care for their elderly parents. The unmarried sister, however, could not escape the duty to care by pointing to her own projects, personal or professional.

Williams (1985) argued that personal projects—those that define a person's self-identity—should override many moral obligations. From this perspective, no person should be expected to give up those projects and interests central to his or her image of self. The traditional view, of course, was that women—all women—are defined by their capacity and instinct to care. Because it was thought that women *want* to care, that it is their nature to care, any woman who resisted the caregiving role was thought to be "unnatural" (Reverby 1987; Rossiter 1982). In many circles, even professional ones, this belief persists, and women are routinely asked to take responsibilities from which men are excused.

Another aspect of this tradition is equally pernicious. Because it was thought that any woman could provide nursing and child care, all those tasks associated with direct bodily care have been devalued. Nursing has experienced a long struggle to achieve status as a semi-profession (Etzioni 1969; Noddings 1990), and even today, early childhood educators are paid very poorly in comparison with elementary and secondary teachers. A quite understandable temptation arises, then, for a financially beleaguered society: Why not hire inexpensive home care workers who will perform tasks in homes for a fraction of the cost that would be charged by professionals in hospitals? Here our society faces a genuine dilemma. On the one hand, costs must be contained, and they can be; on the other hand, cost containment must not induce a new round of exploitation and oppression. Including the concerns of caregivers in our analysis will not in itself resolve the dilemma, but it will help us avoid some traditional errors.

As more women are identified by their professional or occupational choices, a worry arises that women who have chosen homemaking as their main occupation will be further exploited. It is often thought that a female homemaker should contribute her own labor because she is not a wage earner, and even women who earn a small wage outside the home are expected to give up their unprofitable work to provide direct care. A man in the latter situation would rarely experience such an expectation. Women in traditionally male occupations often suffer double castigation—first, for messing about in men's work, and second, for being unwilling to give it up when a family emergency arises.

In considering home care, the caregiver's full load should be analyzed. A professional couple with resources for outside help may be in a better position to provide home care than a full-time homemaker. The latter may have full responsibility for several children, laundry, cleaning, cooking, yard work, and a host of other tasks. If she is middle-aged, she may not be in the best health herself. Young or old, she may not be in a strong position to evaluate her own workload and her capacity to take on yet another physical task. On the positive side, a thorough analysis of this sort may raise the potential caregiver's appraisal of her own worth. Recognition and appreciation may increase her motive energy and help her through a difficult time.

Besides analyzing a caregiver's full load and physical condition, a professional advisor should evaluate the caregiver's attitude toward the particular tasks that must be done. Sometimes a caregiver can cope with difficult technical tasks but dreads some particular part of the daily routine. Mrs. O'Neill had agreed to care for her disabled father at home. She could manage feeding, massage, giving shots, and changing linens, but she simply hated changing his morning diaper. Doing the job made her sick; anticipating it began to interfere with her sleep. This one task pushed the O'Neills to put Mrs. O'Neill's father in a nursing home. If a sympathetic counselor had interviewed Mrs. O'Neill and had assured her that many women find this task repellent—especially for their fathers, who have represented authority in their lives—help might have been hired for just this job. In the case of parents caring for children, parents can often manage everything in the care of a child except that which gives the child most pain. Seeing themselves as their child's protector, they cannot bear this particular aspect of home care (Kohrman 1991). Again, it may be feasible to find help for just these tasks so that parents can continue their otherwise excellent service.

Advisors can also help home care providers with emotional strategies. In a high-tech environment, many health care workers conserve their own emotional strength by concentrating on the machinery and instruments. If this goes too far, conscious patients complain of aloofness and brusqueness. Indeed, many patients prefer home care because of the obvious emotional involvement of their caregivers (Waerness 1984). Further, family caregivers often feel guilty if they focus on the instruments instead of the patient. But it may be helpful for caregivers to know that the strategy reduces emotional strain for some workers and that they should not feel guilty if they need to use it occasionally.

Emotional support for caregivers is essential. Sometimes a support group or counseling is suggested. But caregivers are often stretched thin for time, and many might appreciate the regular visits of a professional caregiver who can give a full range of advice—answer some technical questions, assess the caregiving situation, and provide support for the resident caregiver. (For a good example of this kind of support, see Dominica 1986.)

The home care advisor needs to check on not only the family caregiver's present emotional strength but also the strength of the caregiver's network. Families with strong religious ties often have resources for respite (Hallum 1989). Those without such affiliation may need more help. But even those with longstanding religious connections may find their faith shaken when a family member suffers terribly or when their own lives are disrupted almost beyond recognition (Kushner 1981). Then anger and guilt may be added to physical and emotional exhaustion. Such caregivers need special help.

In this section I have suggested some issues that home care advisors might consider when evaluating the capacities of home care providers. Besides the usual required training, advisors should consider the caregiver's full load of responsibilities, any tasks perceived as overly difficult or emotionally repellent, the caregiver's major projects—particularly those at the core of his or her identity—the caregiver's religious beliefs and whether they are currently providing support or contributing to anger and guilt, and the caregiver's emotional style and whatever coping strategies are compatible with it.

What Are the Positive and Negative Features of the Home's Facilities?

When home care is considered, we must ask not only what the people involved mean to each other but also what their house and each of its rooms mean to them. Sensitive people who run long-term care facilities and hospices know that the comfort and beauty of the surroundings matter to many of their patients. Helen House (Dominica 1986), a hospice for dying children, provides a playroom opening on a beautiful garden, rooms for quiet activities and for noisier ones, and a communal kitchen, where the staff and parents cooperate in cooking and cleaning up. "Light, colour, and space were of prime importance to the design team" (Dominica 1986, p. 117). Most families cannot spend a great deal of money or time on the aesthetic features of the sick room and its surroundings, but they can take these features into consideration.

The room itself must be chosen with care. There must be space for the technical apparatus, of course, and the room should be located so that it is easily accessible to a caregiver who has many other tasks to perform. Often the dining room is chosen because it is downstairs and handy to the kitchen; the patient may also feel less isolated in such a central spot. But if the dining room has always been a family gathering place, a place where the evening meal is shared, it may be a poor choice despite its convenience. Many adults bear lingering resentment toward older relations—long gone—who changed a sunny, happy family place into a smelly, unhappy one. For them, the heart of the home was ripped out when Grandma's bed was moved into the dining room. When the dining room has central meaning for a family, a sunny bedroom upstairs might be a better choice. Then, too, privacy might be more important to the patient than the risk of isolation.

Wherever the patient is located, attention should be given to the aesthetic qualities of the room. People loved to visit Mrs. Traub's young daughter because the room was so inviting. It was the child's room—filled with her hobbies, drawings, and personal possessions. The colorful clutter made it possible for the child to welcome people and share her interests with them. Similarly, an elderly patient who is able to communicate may enjoy familiar photographs, favorite flowers, or a traditional quilt. A loss of self in the patient contributes to fear and dread in both caregivers and visitors. Therefore, the more nearly whole patients can be kept, the easier it may be for caregivers to interact with them.

Whatever space is chosen for home care, it must be kept clean. Again, the caregiver's capacity must be considered. In a hospital, nurses attend to the patient, but they no longer have to scrub the floors, cook the meals, and do the dishes and laundry (Reverby 1987). The family caregiver may have to do all these things. If an arthritic older woman or a mother with several children is the caregiver, she may need help with housekeeping chores. A flexible benefits plan of the sort discussed earlier might provide such help and be less expensive than current alternatives.

In this society, we have not given much thought to the housing needs of families with sick or physically dependent members, and we have given no thought to educating our populace on such matters. Why are houses and apartments not designed with such responsibilities in mind? Properties, too, could be laid out so that small, portable cottages could be added when an elderly parent needs to be close but wishes to remain as independent as possible. (Such a plan has been tried in Canada.) Even condominium and townhouse complexes could be planned to include "dependent apartments" so that semidependent elderly or handicapped persons could live near their families. After World War II, housing developers were often required to build schools for the new neighborhoods they created. Why could we not require high-density developers to provide space for child care, elder care, and sick care? Such arrangements might be considerably less expensive than our current highly specialized, impersonal, and isolated facilities.

Such thinking, to which I return in the final section of this chapter, requires us to think in terms of collective moral obligation, not individual moral obligation. The question with respect to individuals then shifts to how we (the collective) can help them care—what can be done to maintain natural caring. Just as education became a public responsibility in the nineteenth century, so must health care become a public responsibility in the twenty-first century.

Who Is Suffering?

Most accounts of suffering have been patient-centered. Professional attention has been directed to the patient or victim—even, paradoxically, when that person is incapable of suffering. (Suffering is here identified with emotional or psychic pain and, therefore, requires consciousness. For definitions and descriptions of *suffering*, see Starck and McGovern 1992; Taylor and Watson 1989.) Now that technology and medicine have teamed to control physical pain and to prolong biological life, more and more attention is given to what might be called "public suffering," the burdens and deprivations of a society overwhelmed by health costs (Veatch 1977). In ethics, too, we swing from an emphasis on abstract individual rights to one on the collective greatest good. In neither case is the suffering of particular, concrete human beings adequately considered (Benhabib 1987).

In discussions of euthanasia and health rationing, we hear the two extremes. Foot (1978), for example, insisted that euthanasia, if it is to be allowed at all, must be done for the sake of the patient or victim. She realized that in some cases, patients' lives are neither a good nor an evil to them; that is, the patients are incapable of pain or pleasure. Yet she would not consider euthanasia unless "suffering sets in." But genuine suffering may surround the patient. Parents who neglect other children to sit beside a permanently comatose child, adult children who regularly visit an insensate parent, nurses who daily watch the agony of these visitors—all these people are suffering. Shouldn't this suffering be taken into account? In asking and discussing this question, we should not rush to a universal solution, but we should raise the question and answer it affirmatively. The objective is to include all forms of suffering in our discussion.

Some recent plans to control health care costs exhibit an insensitivity to suffering comparable to that encountered in the discussion of euthanasia. A gay man with AIDS recently complained that under a proposed plan, he would be denied a procedure that might make his life more enjoyable on the grounds that he would not live for five more years. Apparently, the procedure fails a cost-effectiveness analysis when applied to those with a short life expectancy. But this man is suffering, and his suffering is increased by the callous way in which his personhood is disregarded. The same society that can entertain such solutions is self-righteously opposed to the merciful killing of those totally incapable of suffering. For a response-to-need orientation to be useful in guiding policy, we must have the courage to listen to cries of need and to reject prescriptions based on highly romanticized and outdated principles.

A third example of our society's inclination to ignore substantial suffering is found in aggressive approaches to saving the lives of profoundly handicapped babies. Saving some such lives not only dooms the infant to a life of pain and, sometimes, humiliation but also assigns parents to many years of near-total sacrifice (Feinberg 1991; Hallum 1989; Veatch 1977). Usually, but not always, it is the mother who gives up work outside the home and most of her personal projects. Often marriages break up under the strain. Both parents and any other children may suffer greatly. To acknowledge this suffering is not to conclude straightaway that all profoundly handicapped infants should be candidates for euthanasia. Solutions should fit the beliefs and capacities of those who will bear the burden. What should be avoided is the seemingly high moral tone that is so easy to project when "saving a life"—a life that will, in fact, call on others to sacrifice theirs.

As we approach the twenty-first century, we will have to ask and answer hard questions. In preparing to discuss these questions intelligently, we must get beyond the unfortunate dichotomy—individual or society—and think in terms of actual human beings. Who is suffering? Why have we so seldom asked this question in the past? Probably, "we" have not asked it because writers and sufferers have been, for the most part, two distinct groups. Now that women are finding their voices, it may be less easy to ignore the suffering of caregivers.

A home care advisor should be sensitive to suffering throughout the network. Does a spouse suffer from lack of companionship? Does a healthy child feel ignored and guilty for feeling so? Have friendships lapsed? Are pets being abused? Sometimes the bystanders' suffering can be relieved by involving them more actively in the patient's care or in some other vital activity of the household. Primary caregivers, even when overworked, need to be reminded that others need their continued care and appreciation. This reminder may free them to give care that is reciprocated and thus more rewarding.

Finally, there are times when the patient should be involved in helping to reduce the suffering of others. On good days, a patient might be able to sort mail, shell peas, draw cats for an appreciative toddler, play checkers with a small boy, or give the family pet some much-needed affection. Caregivers should be helped to overcome guilt and exercise some imagination in this area.

Thoughts for the Next Century

At the beginning of this chapter, I argued that we should put aside the notion of individual moral obligation in favor of one of moral support. The need to do this arises, at least in part, from a critical evaluation of the two main traditional ethics. Kantianism and its host of neoforms have led to a concentration on individual rights, victims, and moral agents. Carried away by the success of rights-talk (Dworkin 1978), we tend to forget that rights are granted and taken away by human beings under various social conditions. Even those rights, such as free speech, that a people hold most precious require new rationales in new times (Graber 1991). Most worrisome is the plain fact that the Kantian ethic of obligation and duty ignores the very conditions that give rise to the demand for rights and that lead people to follow or break the rules they have agreed on.

To insist today that individuals have a moral obligation to care for their children, siblings, or parents invites a debate over the limits of obligation, fairness among those obligated, and renewed attention to the individual rights of agents and victims. Worse, such insistence overlooks the fact that many, perhaps most, people want to care for their loved ones. They need help, not legal coercion or preaching, to do so.

The primary alternative to Kantianism in recent times has been utilitarianism. In utilitarianism, we turn our attention from the individual moral agent to public policy and that which will optimize the ratio of happiness over pain. But now persons lose their individuality and become numbers in faceless classes—the young or old, insured or uninsured, productive or unproductive—and the enormous suffering of a few can be justified by the more enormous collective contentment of the many. Again, utilitarianism—like Kantianism—has effected important social gains, but it will not do if we wish to establish a society in which people are cherished in all their individuality and within their particular relations. Collective obligation has to be aimed not at direct action but at the social conditions that make it possible for people to care for one another.

In this last sense, it does make sense to speak of moral obligation;

that is, it makes sense to say that the public as a collective agent has responsibility for the health and well-being of its citizens. The analogy I used earlier was to public education. But, of course, if we are not careful, this choice can lead back into the thicket of rights and limitations. Just as we ask, How much education must a society make available? we may ask, How much in health services should be made available? to whom? What are the legitimate limits? Who will decide what is meant by "legitimate"?

A better way to respond to the question of which health services should be made available is to say that we will aim to provide whatever people need. This still leaves the theoretical field wide open to the analysis of *need*. But it locates us in the domain of natural caring. This is the way we respond to our children and other loved ones. Sometimes we have to persuade them that they really do not need something they want, and sometimes we have to meet needs by priority, but the ones who express the needs are involved in setting the priorities.

Response to need as the basic orientation in health care policy also points us to analysis in other areas of public policy—in housing, as I noted earlier, and in education. Educational policy, like all of public policy, has long been dominated by Kantian and utilitarian thinking. We urge students to "get an education" so that they can "make it" in life. We insist that everyone has a right to a college education, and whether or not children want it or can profit from it, we cram college preparatory information into as many as will hold still for it (Noddings 1992). With our eyes loftily on a better society, we move children about willy-nilly to achieve racial and ethnic balance, ignoring the needs of particular children for particular kinds of attention.

Using an ethic of care, a response-to-need orientation, educational policymakers would work with policymakers in health care. We would shift the emphasis from the material benefits of education to broader human benefits. Schooling would be aimed at the "good life" construed in terms of both relational and individual development. This is not mad idealism but plain common sense. A recent comprehensive study showed, much to the surprise of the researchers, that students and teachers have very different concerns from researchers and policymakers (IET 1992). Whereas policymakers are concerned about test scores and inducing more students to take math and science, students and teachers are concerned with relations. They long to care and be cared for, to explore questions about what the good life is and how to achieve it.

We could increase the number of people who want to care by

making a life of natural caring a legitimate aim of education. Today students are taught that education will bring them material benefits. It is not surprising, then, that many are unwilling to sacrifice those material benefits to care for others. Indeed, it is surprising that so many still want to care. Our public policies should aim to maintain and enhance the desire and willingness to care. An emphasis on moral obligation, as opposed to one on the richness and joy of relational life, can only promote self-protection and a renewed emphasis on the rights of individuals to pursue material goods, keep them, and even increase them at the expense of a faceless public. We can do better.

This chapter has attempted an analysis of the factors that should be taken into account when high-tech home care is considered. It has also attempted a prolegomena of sorts for public policy based on an ethic of care and response to need. As such, it suggests an alternative to the traditional approaches derived from Kantian and utilitarian ethics.

REFERENCES

Abel, E. R. 1991. *Who Cares for the Elderly?: Public Policy and the Experience of Adult Daughters.* Philadelphia: Temple University Press.

Benhabib, S. 1987. The generalized and the concrete other. In S. Benhabib and D. Cornell, eds., *Feminism as Critique,* pp. 77–95. Minneapolis: University of Minnesota Press.

Callahan, D. 1985. What do children owe elderly parents? *Hastings Center Report* 15:32–37.

Crystal, S., Fleming, C., Beck, P., and Smolka, G., eds. 1987. *The Management of Homecare Services.* New York: Springer.

Dominica, F. 1986. The dying child: A hospice for children. In R. Spilling, ed., *Terminal Care at Home,* pp. 113–30. Oxford: Oxford University Press.

Dworkin, R. M. 1978. *Taking Rights Seriously.* London: Duckworth.

Etzioni, A., ed. 1969. *The Semi-professions and Their Organization: Teachers, Nurses, and Social Workers.* New York: Free Press.

Feinberg, E. A. 1991. Ethical issues. In M. J., Mehlman, and S. J. Youngner, eds., *Delivering High Technology Home Care,* pp. 84–124. New York: Springer.

Foot, P. 1978. *Virtues and Vices.* Berkeley: University of California Press.

Graber, M. 1991. *Transforming Free Speech.* Berkeley: University of California Press.

Gubrium, J. F. 1991. *The Mosaic of Care: Frail Elderly and Their Families.* New York: Springer.

Hallum, A. 1989. An exploratory study of the impact on parents of caring for a physically dependent, severely disabled adult-age child at home. Ph.D. diss., Stanford University.

Institute for Education in Transformation (IET). 1992. *Voices from the Inside*. Claremont, Calif.: Claremont Graduate School.

Kohrman, A. H. 1991. Psychological Issues. In M. J., Mehlman, and S. J. Youngner, eds., *Delivering High Technology Home Care*, pp. 160–78. New York: Springer.

Kushner, H. 1981. *When Bad Things Happen to Good People*. New York: Schocken Books.

McNulty, E. G., and Dann, M. S. 1985. *The Dilemma of Caring*. Springfield, Ill.: Charles C. Thomas.

Noddings, N. 1984. *Caring: A Feminine Approach to Ethics and Moral Education*. Berkeley: University of California Press.

——. 1990. Feminist critiques in the professions. In C. B. Cazden, ed., *Review of Research in Education* 16:343–424.

——. 1992. *The Challenge to Care in Schools*. New York: Teachers College Press.

Reverby, S. 1987. *Ordered to Care*. Cambridge: Cambridge University Press.

Rossiter, M. W. 1982. *Women Scientists in America: Struggles and Strategies to 1940*. Baltimore: Johns Hopkins University Press.

Silverstone, B., and Hyman, H. K. 1976. *You and Your Aging Parent*. New York: Pantheon Books.

Sommers, T., and Shields, L. 1987. *Women Take Care*. Gainesville, Fla.: Triad.

Starck, P., and McGovern, J. P., eds. 1992. *The Hidden Dimension of Illness: Human Suffering*. New York: National League for Nursing.

Taylor, R. L., and Watson, J., eds. 1989. *They Shall Not Hurt*. Boulder, Colo.: Colorado Associated University Press.

U.S. Congress, Office of Technology Assessment (OTA). 1987. *Technology-dependent Children: Hospital v. Home Care. A Technical Memorandum*. OTA-5M-H-38. Washington, D.C.: U.S. Government Printing Office.

Veatch, R. M. 1977. *Case Studies in Medical Ethics*. Cambridge, Mass.: Harvard University Press.

Waerness, K. 1984. The rationality of caring. *Economic and Industrial Democracy* 5:185–212.

Weil, S. 1977. Reflections on the right use of school studies with a view to the love of God. In G. Panichas, ed., *Simone Weil Reader*, pp. 44–52. Mt. Kisco, N.Y.: Mayer Bell Limited.

Williams, B. 1985. *Ethics and the Limits of Philosophy*. Cambridge, Mass.: Harvard University Press.

10. Transforming Homes and Hospitals

William Ruddick, Ph.D.

Under financial pressure, hospitals are discharging patients "quicker and sicker" into the care of family members or professional home care attendants. Miniaturized or simplified ventilators, drug- and nutrition-infusion devices, various monitors, and other hospital equipment are making this shift from hospital to home feasible, even for seriously dependent patients. How desirable is this shift?

The question may seem perverse. Surely, most patients welcome early hospital discharge, and for good reason. Home is commonly conceived and experienced as a place of security, comfort, privacy, and liberty to be oneself. By contrast, the hospital is often thought of and experienced as a place of insecurity, discomfort, intrusion, and demands for compliance and conformity. The evidence for this contrast is abundant and various: in hospitals, patients get round-the-clock examinations, secondary ("nosocomial") infections, and Jell-O; at home, patients enjoy more sleep, more physical activity, and weight gains (Rossman 1988).

But is this contrast too sharply drawn? How might these stereotypes distort our assessment of the transfer of hospital equipment and care to a patient's home? As with most contrasts, there are notable exceptions—namely, homes with few homelike virtues and hospitals with various domestic amenities. But there are, I think, more general troubles with this stark contrast between home and hospital. Most importantly for assessments of hospital-to-home transfers, it ignores the transformations that illness often makes in family life and home. For example, illnesses and treatments can make familiar domestic settings alien, or they can confuse family roles and foster mutual deception, detachment, and resentment, even (or especially) in well-ordered families. Given such transformations, hospitals may often allow patients greater autonomy than home and may better preserve family relationships than would home care—contrary to common assumption. If so, then the current domestication of care for seriously ill patients may be morally questionable in ways the stereotypes of home and hospital obscure.

To explore these paradoxical possibilities, I first examine the contrast between home and hospital, then take up paternalism and autonomy in home and hospital, and finally remark on reasons for choosing not to die at home. Taken together, these reflections suggest that the very features of home and family life that invite hospital-to-home transfers are threatened by those transfers.

Stereotypes of Home and Hospital

In a view reflected in law, poetry, and clichés, home is commonly taken to be a refuge, castle, haven, or nest. (Sir Edward Coke (17th c.): "One's home is the safest refuge to everyone, . . . for a man's house is his castle, *et domus sua cuique tutissimum refugium*.)" As a secure place, home is free from unwelcome intrusions or supervision. As a refuge, it allows ready access, a place to which we can return at will. Witness Robert Frost's oft-quoted farmer in "Death of a Hired Man" as he watches a former worker returning across a field: "Home is the place where, when you have to go there, / They have to take you in." The farmer's wife responds, "I should have called it / Something you somehow haven't to deserve."

In recent centuries, home is also a place of comfort and intimacy (Rybczynski 1986). It is where we can be at ease, without public personae or pressures to conform to social norms. Indeed, for many people, home is where they feel most truly themselves, the very center of their lives, closest relationships, and most intense emotions. As such, home is their natural or, in Aristotelian terms, their "telic place" where mature selves are realized and revealed.

This ideal clearly best fits middle-class family and living conditions. Too few rooms or too many children, close neighbors, or servants would seem to defeat this ideal, and yet it is widely shared, even by solitary dwellers and collective groups. For example, urban "homeless" people recreate minimal homes out of scrap materials in abandoned railway tunnels, concealed bridge niches, and other secure, sheltered spaces (Brown 1993). People attracted to a simpler life in the wild or on the highway may reject furniture or fixed abodes but nonetheless look for security, access, personal accommodation, however idiosyncratically defined. One writer, once free of her children, no longer cared about comfortable furnishings; all she required of her home, apart from secure doors, was a roof to keep out wind and rain—and most importantly, "the terrifying sight of the infinite night sky" (Cantwell 1990). For people whose identity and chosen life are strongly communal, home may have few, if any, private spaces. In the army, convent, or kibbutz, privacy may be provided primarily by the gates or walls that restrict the entry or gaze of outsiders.

As with all ideals, this concept of home poses practical problems, even for the most fortunate middle-class families. Security, comfort, and personal accommodations require regular thought and effort, especially for homes with children and other dependent residents. It is a daunting task to provide people of such various ages, needs, and desires with equitable degrees of these defining domestic desiderata. It requires the skill of a wise (home) economist, as well as the sacrifices of an altruist. In the role of designated "homemaker," women have often had to forego the very virtues of home they provide for others. (As George Bernard Shaw put it, "A man's castle is his daughters' workhouse and his wife's prison.") This taxing and often unappreciated work may lead homemakers to neglect or abuse their dependents and resentfully to fight with those cohabitants who work outside the home, even if they thereby provide material support. In such cases, even minimal security may require outsiders to breach the privacy that allows various abuses to occur.

Despite such complexities and abuses, many homes do approximate this ideal. So, too, perhaps do other residences, including some chronic care hospitals. But acute care hospitals are thought of, and often experienced, as the very antithesis of home—full of discomforts, risks, talkative roommates, depersonalizing routines, impersonal and hurried staff, and so on. As in the army, individual concerns are ignored or suppressed in the interests of maintaining institutional order and effectively fighting the enemy (here, disease and death). In short, hospitals would seem to be the very paradigm of uncongenial, inhospitable places. From a hospital bed, even a woefully inadequate home can seem inviting.

These contrasting stereotypes, however, too often belie the facts and betray patients' hopes: hospitals may prove more hospitable and homelike than some patients' homes. I have in mind not just those homes whose conditions contribute to disease, injury, or exhaustion. More generally, illness and treatment can transform even spacious quarters and caring family relationships into hospital-like conditions. Rooms may lose their comforting familiarity, and families may lose their familial intimacies and mutual trust.

Domestic Paternalism and Abuses

The most paradoxical home-hospital reversals are in matters of patients' liberties and privacy. It is tempting to assume that home provides patients with greater control over their lives than do hospitals (Collopy, Dubler, and Zuckerman 1990). But this is often not so. For example, patients may have a greater sense of privacy in a hospital, not less. In a hospital, otherwise highly personal matters may be depersonalized or impersonalized. Despite constant hospital traffic and intrusions, patients may quickly become used to exposing their bodies or bowel movements to professional caretakers. Such indifference may be harder to achieve with family intimates, especially in rooms once private but now invaded at will by family and professional caregivers. As city dwellers know, privacy is often less a matter of solitude than of anonymity and mutually acceptable indifference in public places.

Patients often complain about being treated impersonally, as "mere cases." But this depersonalization has a further benefit. As "mere cases," hospital patients are allowed to focus entirely on and fully express their symptoms and complaints. To be sure, hospital patients are expected to have some consideration for fellow patients and the staff. But even if they must moderate their groans or complaints, especially at night, patients are less constrained than when with friends and relatives. During visiting hours, for example, patients are under social and moral pressures to conceal or minimize their suffering and fears. After visiting hours, they may revert to their shrunken, self-absorbed world of illness. They can once again be themselves—their sick selves.

At home, however, visiting hours are continuous. Not only must patients keep up continuous pretenses for the sake of worried children, spouses, and friends but also they may be under pressure to improve on their former grumpy, pessimistic, or cynical ways. Admittedly, hospital decorum dictates optimistic and cheerful demeanor of patients as well as staff, but patients are allowed more lapses than at home.

Moreover, home patients may be expected to resume at least some family responsibilities and routines from which hospitalization temporarily freed them. At home it is difficult for a patient to be just a patient, rather than a husband-patient or mother-patient. On the other hand, home patients may not be allowed to resume prior responsibilities they might wish to reclaim along with their prior role in family life. One or more family members may welcome the chance to exercise controlling care, especially on behalf of someone who has previously cared for them. And, by way of justifying this assumption of responsibilities, they may regard home patients as more incapable or incompetent than they are. Indeed, family members may regard patients as childlike.

To so regard anyone we wish to help is tempting. We respond most directly to the needs of children, confident of our ability, right, and responsibility to impose help if necessary. Accordingly, it is tempting to cast anyone we wish to help as childlike, dependent on us for the very assistance that we in our adult skills and knowledge of the world can effectively provide.

This tendency may explain why physicians and nurses often maintain that all seriously ill people revert to childlike dependencies and attitudes. This is no doubt an exaggeration, especially for hospital patients. Adults may react against institutional regimens with adolescent rebellion or merely resentful obstinacy, but neither response is the kind of regression that justifies paternalistic action by hospital staff.

There may, however, be a greater tendency to regression at home. In hospital rooms with other patients, patients may be kept from regression by the stimulus of adult company and social pressure to behave in adult ways among relative strangers. By contrast, home patients without such social stimulus and constraint may lapse into ways and moods learned during childhood illness. Homes are the natural sites and schools for paternalistic practices. Children, especially when ill, are subject to coercion, deception, insincere optimism, and the other arts parents use to manipulate or skirt children's desires in order to serve their interests. While playing their assigned juvenile part (often knowingly or even willingly), children learn these paternalistic skills and in turn use them on younger siblings, grandparents with dementia, and even ill parents themselves. To so act gives a child something of adult status; hence, even if living with a chronically ill parent forces a child "to grow up fast," this may not be an altogether unwelcome demand.

In short, "juvenilistic regression" is a tempting condition of home life for seriously ill patients—a condition that professional home care workers may foster or oppose. Out of principle and practice, they may see themselves as champions of their patients' autonomy against family paternalists. On the other hand, they may become more controlling than hospitals allow. In closer contact with home patients, nurses may make more confident judgments of a patient's best interests than they do in a hospital. Also they may be more subject to family requests (for example, to withhold bad news from a patient or to collude in frank deception). Moreover, there are no patient advocates present in the home to ensure patients' rights.

How serious is this domestic paternalism by family and professionals? Paternalism is not in itself objectionable: to treat someone as a child is not necessarily harmful or insulting. Indeed, when ill, we may welcome such parental concern and confidence in our caretakers. If most professional caregivers were like ideal mothers or fathers—powerful, loving, devoted, knowledgeable of us and of the world—would patients or their families need or want a large or continuous role in health care decisions? I think not.

Paternalism becomes a problem when, as in most hospitals, there is a scarcity of such devoted, careful caregivers. In institutions staffed by overworked students, nurses, and residents tending too many patients with various maladies and native languages, patients need the protection of enforceable rights. But in a home, our chances of having devoted caretakers, family or professional nurses, are far greater.

On the other hand, like any vulnerable, dependent person, a patient—whether in a hospital or at home—is subject to the anger, impatience, resentment, and sadomasochistic exercises of power by caregivers, professional or familial. The psychodynamics of family relationships and the privacy of homes may, in fact, increase the risks of such abuse. How then should home patients be protected? How should safeguards be formulated? Is some current Hospital Patients' Bill of Rights a model?

Some of those hospital rights are clearly unnecessary at home—especially those meant to protect patients against the often anonymous, diffuse, hurried care in large hospitals (for example, the right to respectful, compassionate care, or to know the name of the physician directing one's care, or to complain to a patient advocate). Other rights (for example, to informed consent) seem less pressing for home patients who are convalescing or stabilized by a steady therapeutic regimen. Perhaps the most important would be the right to refuse treatment, especially life-sustaining treatment. Unlike hospital patients who often face unfamiliar treatments with uncertain outcomes, chronically ill or dying patients may know all too well what continuing treatment, such as kidney dialysis or mechanical respiration, involves, and yet may be intimidated by intimate caretakers from even raising the issue of discontinuance. A recognized right to discontinue treatment might at least allow them to express their hesitations about continuing a painful course without the hope of improvement.

This right would be secured by a more general right to leave home for some other place of care or some other place to die—a nursing home, hospital, hospice, friend's residence, or some beloved city or natural place. Hospital patients, if competent, have such exit rights to check themselves out "AMA" (against medical advice). The value of this right is obvious for patients in "total institutions" without their clothes, money, and ready access to unguarded exits.

Exit rights are at least as important for a home patient. Using Albert Hirschman's notion of "exit voice," certain feminist theories (Gilligan 1986; Okin 1989) have stressed the value, especially for weaker members of a family or other small collectives, of knowing that one can leave. Otherwise, membership is coercive, imprisoning, or destructive of individual identity. Since chronic or terminal illness may already undermine a person's identity, an exit right would be even more important than in normal domestic circumstances.

Threats to personal identity are threats to autonomy, as are the threats to privacy and maturity mentioned above. The meaning and issue of patient autonomy are, I think, too complex to address here. It is enough to note that the liberty to leave home, when sick or ill, may be a necessary condition for the autonomy of both a patient and those family members who have the responsibilities of care thrust on them, often willy-nilly.

Whether a patient can exercise an exit right will depend, of course, on what alternatives are available. Since hospitals and insurers have strong financial interests in moving patients from hospital to home, they are not likely to support the reverse right of patients to transfer at will from home to hospital, or even to nursing homes or hospices. Whether the health care reforms now debated (in 1995) will make alternatives to home care more available is not clear.

Transformations of Home and Patient

Paternalistic control and domestic abuses aside, patients may have other reasons for wanting to leave home for an alternative place of treatment. Contrary to stereotype or initial desires, patients may find that their homes are not as hospitable as they expected or hoped. Illness may produce unexpected changes, not just in family relationships but in the very experience of familiar home spaces. Unlocked or open doors that diminish privacy are just one of the ways in which rooms are transformed by illness and therapeutic equipment. Fever may give walls, windows, or closets a menacing aspect. (I still recall with a shudder the collapsing walls of my childhood chickenpox fevers). Familiar colors and sounds may become abrasive, stairs too steep, shelves too high, rugs treacherous.

Likewise, any physical changes (drawn curtains, rented hospital beds and bathtub rails) may transform a former place of rest and pleasure into confining, repugnant clinical spaces, not only for a patient but also for cohabitants who continue to share those altered spaces, often resentfully. Even if there is a spare room for the home patient and medical equipment, adjacent rooms and their uses may have to be altered: kitchen noises and odors may disturb a patient and have to be minimized; so, too, conversation, music, or television. Obviously, it cannot be assumed that a patient's home, so transformed, remains the familiar, secure, or welcome place it may have been earlier, for either patients or their families.

These transformations of experienced space may be part of a related change of a patient's sense of self. I wrote above of a hospital patient's "sick self." Our sense of self often changes with place, especially with place of residence. In many cases, to return home is to renew or regain the old sense of self, but if illness produces serious and permanent changes of ability, desire, or character, that old sense of self may not be gained by going home. This is especially true if the illness or loss transforms the home. Think, for example, how permanent paraplegia would alter both the sense of one's self and the sense of home, especially if home had been one's defining, natural or "telic" place.

In short, there are two respects in which going home may become conceptually problematic. Given the transformative effects of illness and medical equipment, what was home may no longer be home. And, given the impact of illness on family relationships mentioned above and on other defining features of personal identity, the person who comes home from the hospital may not be the person who left home for the hospital. "You can't go home again" has a special aptness here (Rubinstein 1990). If these changes are fully appreciated or anticipated, some patients may be reluctant to leave the hospital, despite the usual general desire for home. Correlatively, families may resist a patient's return for similar reasons. Apart from the added burden of care, the transformation of home and the ill relative may be experienced as a double, alienating loss of both home and family.

When homes cannot encompass the demands of illness or therapy, family feeling and relationships may be best maintained at a distance, with regular, even if inconvenient, trips to a hospital or nursing home. When serious or chronic illness cancels both the desire to go home and the presumption of ready access that defines home, hospitals may paradoxically become a preferable home away from a home that no longer has the comforts and familiarity and welcome access of home; hospitals or other clinical facilities may provide better home care than a patient's family home.

Home Care Elsewhere

Is "home care in a hospital" an oxymoron? No more so than is "home cooking at a restaurant." Indeed, with the appropriate size, fare, ambiance, clientele, chef, and waiters, a restaurant might be a better source of home cooking than many homes. (Microwaved frozen dinners quickly served and eaten provide little competition.) Is hospital home care equally possible, or would the term "home hospital" be as misleading as the term "nursing home" often is?

Some hospitals are trying to become more homelike. Newly built wings allow family members to live in and help care for convalescent patients (for example, the Cooperative Care unit at New York University Medical Center). Other hospitals (such as Beth Israel, New York) have refitted floors with family rooms, patient microwave kitchens, soft lighting, and home furnishings. Hospital carts and equipment are kept out of sight, hours of testing are limited, meal and medication schedules are flexible, and patients are encouraged to read and talk to nurses and a pharmacist about their illnesses and therapies. "Care companions" and children are welcome visitors. Although this program (the "Planetree Program," after Hippocrates's site of healing) is meant to prepare patients for better and less anxious self-care and home care, these special wings are not meant for convalescing patients alone. A full range of patients is randomly assigned to these homelike quarters, even "step down" transfers from intensive care units and terminally ill patients who prefer these redesigned wings to hospice units.

Even if able to care for themselves at home, some patients will prefer these homelike hospital accommodations to their own residences. Indeed, for chronically ill homeless people, hospitals are their only homes, however Spartan, public, and prisonlike they may be. These new amenities would make hospitals even more attractive alternatives to shelters or the streets.

No doubt skeptics or opponents of homelike conversions will want to count the danger of lingering patients as an added cost, along with the additional time nurses or physicians spend educating patients and their care companions. Advocates of hospital domestication and greater roles for nurses and patients will, by contrast, stress the savings that better-educated and confident patients will generate. Some patients may leave these special units sooner, confident that they and their care partners can cope at home. Moreover, patients trained in self-care may be less likely to make anxious mistakes at home or to think that they have made mistakes that require rehospitalization for correction.

Although cost-effective assessments will, as usual, reflect rather than determine prior judgments of the reforms in question, there are at least two likely points of agreement between advocates and opponents. The usual rationales given for differential treatment of rich and poor will be invoked no doubt to favor reforms in hospitals with a primarily privately insured patient population. ("Poorer patients, we may assume, will be less educable, have fewer responsible care companions," etc.) Second, as Arno, Bonnuck, and Padgug note in chapter 13 of this volume, cost-effective assessments by economists tend to ignore the costs in time, labor, and opportunities of unpaid home workers. Accordingly, care companions are likely to be ignored by both sides in economic disputes about domesticating even private hospitals.

Home and Hospital Deaths

A domestic ambiance has, of course, been the aim of the hospice movement from the start. But as places for terminally ill patients, hospices are probably not a model for general homelike facilities: where and how one dies often create special needs and desires.

Once death is imminent, people often insist on going home to die to be surrounded by family. Even if a hospital allows families to tend a dying relative day and night, they tend to remain visitors who are subject to staff permission and supervision. Moreover, hospitals rarely allow expressions of full family feelings of grief, rage, and love. And for people whose family has been the defining center of their lives, home may seem the only appropriate site for the conclusion to that life.

A historian of obstetrics compared hospital and home births thus: with home delivery, "medicine is a guest in the house of woman, rather than in the hospital, where woman is a guest in the house of medicine" (Arney 1982, p. 213). Dying at home promises many of the same benefits as giving birth at home. There are familiar surroundings and loving, attentive family. Even if there is somewhat greater risk of complication, there is the promise of more patient control of the character of events. Like home births, home deaths are family events, not institutional events (Rothman 1982). In the hospital, even the most sympathetic nurses and residents are institutional officials used to directing matters. In homes, medical attendants are, like chameleons, pressed to assume the local coloration of family or guests. More generally, home deaths may support the hope for more personal, biographically appropriate timing and conditions than hospital deaths. These are the individualized "good deaths" of some recent discussions of euthanasia (Brody 1992; Rachels 1986).

Once again, however, we must guard against simplistic assumptions about home's comforts and opportunities, as well as about hospital's asperities and restrictions. Many patients die from medical conditions that allow little control or personal fine-tuning (Nuland 1994). Even when there are such options, hospitals may be preferable: dying is often agonizing or messy, and consequently patients may prefer the help of impersonal professionals to that of family members—for reasons related to the greater hospital privacy cited above.

For some patients there may be more subtle considerations, related to their conceptions of home and the lingering effects of home deaths, on family survivors who continue to live there. When a patient recovers from an illness, sick room transformations are usually reversible: rented hospital equipment is returned, medicines are jettisoned, and premorbid activities are resumed. But with a home death, mourning family members may find it difficult to undertake such reversions. Removing all physical traces of a last illness may seem disrespectful; hence a home or room may retain its hospital aura. Even if undertaken, these changes may not attenuate vivid memories of an occupant's dying and death.

In some cultures, those memories are given metaphysical substance: places of death are invested with the lingering spirits of people who have suffered and died there. Even in cultures without belief in local postmortem spirits, death beds or death rooms may continue to be strong reminders of those deaths, even after renovation. (For me, the rooms in which my father and a grandmother died were permanently sepulchral.) I can imagine place-sensitive persons choosing to die in a place outside the home so that survivors will not find their dwelling encumbered by death or such semishades.

There may be legal complications of home deaths as well. Although patients may more easily control the means and time of their deaths at home, in so doing they put their families and physicians at legal risk. In a notable case of assisted suicide, a patient with fatal leukemia timed her death with barbiturates prescribed by her sympathetic physician. But to protect her family and himself from legal inquiry, he had to falsify the cause of death (Quill 1991). Such concerns drive some patients to seek aid in dying far from home, often in bleak circumstances (Kevorkian 1991).

Should patients be legally enabled to die at home with family and physician assistance? Support for legalization would be greater but for fears of unwitting and undetectable abuse. Opponents claim that home patients would feel under pressure to spare their families further burdens of care by means of an early death, however devoted their caretakers may be. Moreover, self-deceived or unscrupulous family members might foster such feelings and too readily accede to requests for death assistance. Such abuses would, critics claim, be very hard to prevent or detect, especially in patients' homes.

In hospitals or hospices such feelings and subtle coercions could be lessened. Financial concerns aside, families would be less burdened and hence would have less reason to foster feelings of guilt in a lingering family member, unwittingly or otherwise. Likewise, patients would have less reason to have such feelings and make such requests. Accordingly, we should expect fewer requests for assisted dying in hospice or hospital than in the home—again, financial concerns aside. Moreover, such requests could be more carefully assessed, deferred, or acted upon in a hospital or hospice. And, contrary to some claims about death assistance being contrary to the "mission of medicine," physicians have long given aid of one sort or another in dying, especially in hospitals where life-support is so elaborate and its gradual discontinuance undramatic but predictably effective in hastening death.

Of course, we cannot set financial considerations aside. Since they are a principal cause of moving patients with equipment into the home, financial considerations will keep them from readily returning to the hospital or from spending much time in a hospice. Hence, if patients are to have legally permissible control over their dying, ways must be found to reduce the potential home abuses cited above. Whether the Dutch or Germans have found such ways is subject to debate (Battin 1992). Whether the Oregonians, in implementing a recent referendum in favor of physician-assisted suicide, will do better is subject to speculation.

A final word about the irrelevance of these reflections for two groups of people without homes to which they can be transferred. Having outlived spouses and lived alone, or in communal residences with medical supervision, the elderly may have no place that feels like home. Even the homes of grown children eager to take them in may not be adequate home-substitutes. As for the increasing number of "homeless" people, dying at home is an idle thought. Even if Constitutional lawyers can count cardboard boxes in a tunnel or bridge abutment as a home protected against unwarranted police intrusion, hospital physicians and social workers cannot. For such homeless people, hospitals may be the only place to go to die. Ironically, current urban social conditions are forcing hospitals to revert in part to their premodern role as charnel houses for the poor.

These thoughts may be biased more than I realize by own limited experiences of home and of hospital care and deaths. My home and family life has been strikingly traditional, my hospital stays short and unremarkable, and so, too, the dying and deaths of my parents. Nonetheless, I hope that these reflections provide some reason to question initial enthusiasm for the transfer of hospital equipment and care into the home.

ACKNOWLEDGMENTS

This chapter has been much improved by comments from John Arras, Lauren Bryant, James Dwyer, Frances Kamm, Nancy McKenzie, James Lindemann Nelson, Amèlie Rorty, Sara Ruddick, Ruth Sidel, Victor Sidel, and Arthur Zitrin.

REFERENCES

Arney, W. R. 1982. *Power and the Profession of Obstetrics.* Chicago: University of Chicago Press.

Battin, M. 1992. Assisted suicide: Lessons from Germany. *Hastings Center Report* 22:44–51.

Brody, H. 1992. Assisted death: A compassionate response to a medical failure. *New England Journal of Medicine,* 327:1384–88.

Brown, P. 1993. The architecture of those called homeless. *New York Times,* 28 March, A1.

Cantwell, M. 1990. Close to home. *New York Times,* 23 August, C2.

Coke, E. 17th c. *Third Institute.*

Collopy, B., Dubler, N., and Zuckerman, C. 1990. The ethics of home care: Autonomy and accommodation. *Hastings Center Report* 20:2, suppl., p. 1.

Gilligan, C. 1986. Exit-voice dilemmas in adolescent development. In A. Foxley, M. McPherson, and G. O'Donnell, eds. *Development, Democracy and the Art of Trespassing,* p. 283. Notre Dame, Ind.: University of Notre Dame Press.

Kevorkian, J. 1991. *Prescription: Medicide,* chap. 15. Buffalo, N.Y.: Prometheus Books.

Nuland, S. 1994. *How We Die: Reflections on Life's Final Chapter.* New York: Knopf.

Okin, S. 1989. *Justice, Gender, and the Family.* New York: Basic Books.

Quill, T. 1991. Death and dignity: A case of individualized decision making. *New England Journal of Medicine*, 324:691–94.

Rachels, J. 1986. *The End of Life: Euthanasia and Morality*. New York: Oxford University Press.

Rossman, I. 1988. The geriatrician and the homebound patient. *Journal of the American Geriatrics Society* 36:348–54.

Rothman, B. 1982. *Giving Birth: Alternatives in Childbirth*. New York: Penguin Books.

Rubinstein, R. L. 1990. Culture and disorder in the home care experience: The home as sickroom. In J. Gubrium, and A. Sankar, eds., *The Home Care Experience*. Newbury Park, Calif.: Sage Publications.

Rybczynski, W. 1986. *Home: A Short History of an Idea*. New York: Viking Penguin.

11. Problems and Protocols for Dying at Home in a High-Tech Environment

Marshall B. Kapp, J.D., M.P.H.

People died at home thirty years ago and few members of the public or the health professions gave that natural phenomenon much thought. As the technological capabilities of modern medicine have advanced (U.S. Congress, OTA 1987), however, the locus of life's ending has changed for many to institutional settings.

Ironically, we are beginning to come full circle. Home care is no longer simply custodial. Modern technology enables us to medically treat many patients at home who earlier would have needed to receive treatment in the hospital (Steel 1991). At the same time, an increasing number of people wish to, and believe they can, exercise personal control over that technology better in the home setting than as inpatients at a health care institution. The President's Commission (1983, p. 103) noted, "[Because] many people wish to die at home in familiar surroundings and, in many cases, hospitals discharge terminally or irreversibly-ill patients . . . medical care in the home, especially for terminally and irreversibly ill patients, is increasing."

The advent of high-tech home care for dying persons raises special ethical and legal concerns, as home moves from a place where treatment decisions made elsewhere are carried out to a site where decision making itself happens. These concerns are outlined in this chapter.

Case 1

Mr. Fisher is a 70-year-old smoker with advanced lung cancer, diagnosed a year prior, with a life expectancy of a few months. He is able to make decisions about his medical treatment and has not been adjudicated otherwise. His physicians have communicated clearly and honestly with

him. Mr. Fisher is a widower who lived alone until his last hospitalization. Upon discharge, he moved into the home of his daughter (an only
child) and her family. She does not work outside the home, and she and
the other family members provide Mr. Fisher with substantial informal
caregiving. Mr. Fisher receives a pension and is eligible for Medicare.
Arrangements have been made for the Acme Home Health Agency, a
private, nonprofit, Medicare-certified organization, to come into the
home daily to provide health-related services to Mr. Fisher. These services include an infusion pump for pain control and antibiotics for his
frequent infections.

Mr. Fisher is concerned about the trajectory of his decline and
dying over the next several months and wants to maintain as much
control as possible over, and dignity and comfort during, his final
days. Mr. Fisher should be supported and encouraged to think
through and express his preferences regarding various life-sustaining
medical interventions (probably mechanical ventilation, cardiopulmonary resuscitation, antibiotics, and artificial nutrition) in a clear
and timely manner.

In any setting, the role of the patient's health care providers in
initiating and participating in dialogue concerning treatment values
and preferences is essential. The patient's home ought to present an
especially nonthreatening, congenial (from the patient's perspective)
setting for conducting such a sensitive dialogue.

In an interactive relationship, contingencies should be discussed
with a mentally capable patient like Mr. Fisher in a dialogue that
proceeds over a period of time rather than a discussion that begins
and shortly thereafter ends at a single point. The American Medical
Association's (AMA) home care guidelines (1992, p. 15) recommend
that physicians talk with the patient about "participation in treatment decisions and wishes concerning rehospitalization, resuscitation, and use of various medical technologies." Since Mr. Fisher is
capable of making decisions, his family theoretically should be privy
to confidential information and participate in treatment discussions
only to the extent that he authorizes. However, since he lives with
his family and relies on them for informal caregiving, he probably
wants their active participation in treatment discussions; as a practical matter, he probably could not prevent their involvement in this
phase of treatment planning. If the family were supporting Mr.
Fisher's care financially as well, its claim to participation in treatment
decisions would be even stronger ethically and more likely practically.

In the context of home care, the interdisciplinary team's involvement in the patient's care plan in assisting the patient and family through an extended series of treatment decisions unfolding over time is underscored (AMA 1992). The nursing literature emphasizes the function of the home care nurse in helping the patient and family understand treatment options and consequences and in listening to their concerns during multiple conversations (Bigler 1990; Brown and Rousseau 1990). Nurses and other members of the interdisciplinary team must be prepared to participate effectively in these discussions, including preparation for referring the patient to sources of legal and other advice beyond the nurse's expertise (Carr 1992).

The conversations about treatment values and preferences among Mr. Fisher, his family, and the interdisciplinary team members should be guided by the agency's written policies and procedures on advance medical directives and medical decision making. As a home care agency certified to participate in Medicare and/or Medicaid, Acme falls under the requirements of the Patient Self-Determination Act (PSDA) enacted as part of the 1990 Omnibus Budget Reconciliation Act (OBRA).* While this federal statute and the implementing regulations promulgated by the U.S. Department of Health and Human Services are not intended to create new substantive patient rights,† they do impose a number of procedural obligations on health care providers.

Acme is commanded, as a condition of receiving federal dollars for its services, to: (*a*) maintain written policies and procedures concerning advance directives; (*b*) provide written information to each adult patient concerning an individual's rights under state law to make decisions concerning such medical care, including the right to accept or refuse medical treatment and the right to formulate, at the individual's option, advance directives and the provider's written policies respecting the implementation of such rights, including a clear and precise statement of limitation if the provider cannot implement an advance directive on the basis of conscience; (*c*) document in the individual's medical record whether or not the individual has executed an advance directive; (*d*) not condition the provision of care or otherwise discriminate against an individual based on whether or not the individual has executed an advance directive; (*e*) ensure compliance with the requirements of state law regarding advance directives; (*f*) provide for staff education concerning its policies and procedures on advance directives; and (*g*) provide for community

---

*Public Law 101–508 (1990), §§ 4206 (Medicare) and 4751 (Medicaid).
† 42 Code of Federal Regulations §489.102.

education regarding advance directives, either directly or in concert with other providers and organizations.

Under the same law, each state must, "acting through a State agency, association, or other private nonprofit entity, develop a written description of the State law (whether statutory or as recognized by the courts of the State) concerning advance directives . . . to be distributed by . . . providers . . . in accordance with the requirements [imposed on providers under the PSDA]."*

The intent of the act is to enhance patient autonomy by facilitating more informed, timely medical decision making, in terms of both the patient's initial selection of a particular provider and the patient's control regarding specific treatments once the provider/patient relationship has been established. In the spirit of the act, even home health agencies that are not legally bound to do so ought ethically to create and share with prospective patients formal organizational policies and procedures regarding medical decision making (Thobaben 1992). Besides serving the interests of patient autonomy and informed decision making, notifying the patient and family prospectively of organizational attitudes, particularly concerning any misgivings about honoring patient or family instructions, and internal dispute resolution procedures should proactively help avoid or mitigate later disagreements about, or disruptions in, the delivery of care and certainly should reduce the likelihood that disputes would be submitted to the courts for resolution.

The imposition of PSDA responsibilities on home care providers has not occurred without controversy. Some home health agencies object to being thrust into an informational role that rightly belongs to the physician as an integral aspect of the physician/patient therapeutic relationship, especially since the physician is the one legally empowered to write the treatment or nontreatment orders for the patient that the home care staff is bound to follow (Dombi 1991). Some physicians, perhaps jealous of their domain, have joined in this criticism. The problem is that many individuals do not have an established, ongoing relationship with a specific primary care physician, and even those who enjoy such a relationship may find the physician reluctant to participate in, let alone initiate, conversation about end-of-life treatment issues, especially well before those issues are directly confronting that particular patient. The proper response to this criticism of the PSDA is not to reduce the informational responsibilities of home care agencies but to encourage physicians to take the initia-

---

*42 Code of Federal Regulations §431.20.

tive in this arena within their medical practices and to influence general health care policy so that every person enjoys an ongoing primary care physician/patient relationship within which meaningful discussions about future treatment preferences and values can take place in advance of crisis.

Additionally, the home care agency's formal policies and procedures should explicitly deal with its relationship with the physicians who attend the agency's patients, defining precisely the respective duties and expectations of the parties (Haddad and Kapp 1991). Formal concurrence with the agency's policies by the attending physician should be made a condition of affiliation with the agency or, if the patient's right to select a personal physician is considered paramount, the patient should at least be informed early of any serious differences in basic attitudes toward advance directives between the agency and the physician. Similarly, the home care agency should have policy provisions regarding, and memoranda of understandings with, other relevant independent contractors who may be involved with patient care and with questions of the use of life-sustaining technology.

A related problem noted with the PSDA is the proliferation of inconsistent organizational policies and procedures that a single home care patient may encounter. Within the continuum of care that many patients and families experience, they may be exposed to an array of hospitals, nursing homes, and home health agencies, each provider with its own set of policies and procedures concerning medical decision making. Patients and families may receive, and become confused and frustrated by, differing and mixed philosophical signals. The problem could be exacerbated if the patient has recently received medical attention in multiple states. It is conceivable that patients and families caught at a very vulnerable moment, when a home care program from which a patient is not expected to leave alive is entered into, may feel intimidated into executing poorly understood or tepidly embraced advance directives as a result of the cumulative, persuasive effect of confusing but powerful information sent from different directions.

The PSDA represents just one piece of the intricate regulatory context within which Acme Home Care Agency, Mr. Fisher, and his family must wend their way toward an acceptable dying scenario (Spiegel 1991). Each state, as a condition of participation in Medicaid, must develop and make available to covered health care providers a written statement of state legislative and judicial policy regarding advance directives and medical decision making. Although certain important ethical principles (such as the right of a mentally capable, informed patient like Mr. Fisher to permit or refuse life-sustaining medical interventions) are entrenched in our jurisprudence, confusing and restrictive legal vagaries may exist among different states or even within a single state on other important details.

Other parts of the regulatory atmosphere consist of state licensure statutes; Medicare Conditions of Participation found in 1987 OBRA amendments* and implementing regulations,† including those on the right to make informed choices regarding treatment;‡ and accreditation from private bodies such as the Community Health Accreditation Program of the National League for Nursing§ and the Joint Commission on Accreditation of Healthcare Organizations‖ (JCAHO 1994). Most states have conscience clauses in their advance directive statutes allowing noncompliance with a patient's treatment wishes on the basis of the provider's philosophical disagreement, as long as the patient has been informed beforehand of this contingency.

Statutes on elder abuse and neglect may lead to criminal and/or civil sanctions against home care agencies for the acts and omissions of the staff (*Caretenders, Inc. v. Commonwealth*, Kentucky Court of Appeals, 21 September 1990). Bayer (1986, p. 55) warned, "If we decentralize the care of the elderly and frail, the possibility of hidden neglect will increase. It will be very difficult to monitor what goes on behind those millions of closed doors. This is the first and preeminent risk associated with the home care movement: Neglect masquerading as more humane care."

Abuse and neglect laws are not intended to inhibit Acme from respecting the choice of Mr. Fisher and his family to forgo aggressive medical intervention in favor of palliative care. It is conceivable, though unlikely, that some outside party might complain to a law-enforcement entity about the situation. While negative repercussions for the family or Acme would be extremely speculative, even their remote specter and the negative accompanying publicity could inhibit certain unduly nervous families and home care agencies.

The free-floating anxiety about malpractice lawsuits that per-

---

*Public Law 100–203, 101 Stat. 1330–67–1330–75, Title IV (Subpart B) (1987).
† 42 Code of Federal Regulations Part 484. Slightly revised final regulations were published at 56 *Federal Register* 32967–32975 (18 July 1991).
‡ 42 Code of Federal Regulations §484.10 (c).
§ 57 *Federal Register* 22273–79 (29 May 1992).
‖ 58 *Federal Register* 35,007–35,017 (30 June 1993).

vades the health care industry cannot be overlooked in any discussion of the delivery of health-related patient services. Besides the systemic barriers that limit the bringing of malpractice actions against professional home care providers generally (Johnson 1991), Acme's conscientious inclusion of Mr. Fisher's family in discussions about his treatment choices, its compliance with its own policies and procedures regarding medical decision making, and its careful documentation of communications and actions form a sensible risk-management strategy that should keep malpractice fears from interfering with ethical conduct in this case.

Questions have been raised about whether the presence of these quality-assurance mechanisms, plus the fact that few home care agencies have developed formal internal mechanisms handling bioethical issues, may lead to more external scrutiny of private agreements to abate certain life-sustaining medical interventions in the home setting. Others have speculated that professionals may fail to probe a patient's refusal of treatment as carefully in the home environment as in a hospital or nursing home, that providers may be more likely to accept the home care patient's purported decision to limit life-sustaining medical interventions at face value (Collopy, Dubler, and Zuckerman 1990). This may be especially objectionable if the patient's decision to forgo life-sustaining treatments is less than truly informed or capable because the patient underestimated and underappreciated the risks and consequences involved, reasoning erroneously that "if I were really sick, I would be in a hospital. I'm all right if I'm at home" (Collopy, Dubler, and Zuckerman 1990, p. 8).

Dubler (1990) argued that a presumption in favor of a patient's right to make such decisions ought to be stronger in the home than in an institution. In judging the capacity to make decisions, she urged, the authenticity of the patient's choice should be afforded more weight than present cognition. Indeed, the familiar and nonthreatening surroundings of home should enhance the patient's cognitive capacities and the ability to make decisions consistent with previously held values and preferences, thereby justifying deference to the patient's spoken choice. Further, it is difficult to conduct many sophisticated diagnostic tests in the patient's home, thereby decreasing the medical certainty with which expected benefits of treatment may be predicted and hence diminishing the authority of any recommendations in favor of aggressive interventions entailing life-sustaining medical technologies (Dubler 1990).

Against this backdrop, what is the proper role for Mr. Fisher's family regarding first, the process of decision making for Mr. Fisher and second, informal caregiving and support for Mr. Fisher in implementing treatment decisions?

Theoretically, for a capable patient like Mr. Fisher, the family's role would be first advising him to the extent that he requested, as he rationally evaluated information communicated to him by the interdisciplinary home care team in the light of his lifetime of accumulated values and preferences, and then supporting him and his choice. More commonly, medical decision making at home is a shared endeavor (Kapp 1991), with the family either giving support to, or placing pressure on, the patient in either direction. When the patient and home care providers disagree about specific treatments, families can make it easier or harder for the professionals to gang up on the patient (Dubler 1990). When a disagreement exists between even a capable patient and the family, family interests in determining the outcome arguably take on ethical significance in proportion to the degree to which the family will pay for and/or provide the care necessary to effectuate the choices reached (Dubler 1992).

This is the crux of the family's role. Mr. Fisher retains decisional autonomy but lacks its executional counterpart (Collopy 1988). He has the right to make choices about medical treatment but depends heavily on his family to care for him as an essential part of fulfilling his decisions.

Mr. Fisher's case approximates the "Rockwellian image of high tech/high touch" described by one author as "the trigenerational family sitting by the hearth with a back-up oxygen tank perched next to the grandfather clock" (Feinberg 1991, p. 95). For real families, the family/patient relationship engendered by the informal caregiving experience will be considerably more complex and difficult.

Feinberg (1991, p. 95) wrote: "The assumptions of high tech home care can be perceived as an assault on the independence and autonomy of the middle-aged adult child of elderly parents. It reverses the pattern of decreasing dependence that is a hallmark of the evolving family system and demands a return to a concept of the original nuclear family as deeply interconnected for the duration of the life of the last surviving parent. High tech home care raises fundamental ethical questions regarding the nature of family relationships [and] the priorities of obligation." In assessing what the family owes to its dependent members (Callahan 1985), we should consider the costs in terms of lost income, leisure and career opportunities, and interaction with other family members.

When the family has taken on caregiving tasks, a question arises about the ethical and legal authority/responsibility to intervene when the family is failing in those tasks to the patient's detriment (Arras 1995). It is unclear when the home care agency would be compelled to cease looking the other way and take action as the patient's advocate, either morally or under statutes for reporting adult abuse and neglect (Collopy, Dubler, and Zuckerman 1990).

Case 2

> Mr. Fisher is incapable of making decisions at the time of his last hospital discharge, although he has not been adjudicated incompetent. However, six months earlier, while capable of making decisions, he executed both an instruction directive stating that no "heroic measures" be used to keep him alive artificially after there was no hope of recovery and a proxy directive naming his daughter as the surrogate decision maker in the event of future incapacity.

In this case, Mr. Fisher's advance directives would be useful in determining his final course of care at home (Connaway 1985). Legislation exists in every state describing the process for executing such directives. "Natural death" laws authorize both living wills or declarations (instruction directives) and durable powers of attorney for health care (proxy directives). Confusion may arise over the interpretation of some state statutes that appear to restrict the prerogatives of mentally capable individuals to direct future treatment in some respects, but the better view is that state legislation may only procedurally effectuate or substantively expand, but may not substantively limit, the constitutional decisional rights that have been recognized in the medical treatment area (Kapp 1992, 1993). Advance medical directives have been used successfully in home care (Markson and Steel 1990).

Another form of prospective directive that might follow from Mr. Fisher's living will, from conversations with the agent under the durable power of attorney, or from earlier conversations between a mentally capable Mr. Fisher and the home health team would be orders written by Mr. Fisher's physician to other providers to refrain from initiating particular interventions. These "Do Not" orders might involve hospitalization, intubation, or other interventions that Mr. Fisher previously indicated a desire to avoid under certain circumstances. Most ethical and legal attention to "Do Not" orders thus far, though, has revolved around cardiopulmonary resuscitation (CPR) (used here as shorthand for an array of basic and advanced cardiac life-support technologies).

In general, there is a legal and ethical presumption in favor of performing CPR on a patient with cardiac arrest. This presumption would be overcome, however, in case 2. Mr. Fisher, while still capable, made an informed decision, supported by his family, to forgo CPR in the event of arrest because the anticipated physical, psychological, and financial burdens to him would outweigh the minimal expected benefit of, at most, a short life extension with poor quality until the next arrest. The experience of home care programs is that few patients or families are reluctant to engage in Do Not Resuscitate (DNR) conversations, and most are thankful when the subject is broached (Havlir, Brown, and Rousseau 1989).

A problem might occur if, when Mr. Fisher arrests at home, his family panics and calls the rescue squad instead of letting Mr. Fisher die. In this common scenario (Loewy 1988), it is standard for the emergency squad to be guided by the normal presumption in favor of rescue intervention and to override family protestations to let the patient die peacefully (Coll and Anderson 1992).

To address this problem and assure that patients' wishes about CPR are honored, emergency medical personnel and other pertinent health care actors (e.g., medical societies, hospital and nursing home associations, home care agencies, and hospices) in many states and localities are working jointly to establish "portable" DNR protocols to confer legal protection on emergency squads for respecting home-based DNR orders while guarding against mistakes that jeopardize patients who want the last ounce of medical technology (Sachs, Miles, and Levin 1991). The content of these policies and procedures varies widely in terms of covered interventions under a prehospital "Do Not" order and the means of documenting and validating the order to withhold. It has been suggested that for withholding CPR at home, specific physician-written DNR orders are preferable to relying exclusively on more global instruction directives, because the latter require too much interpretation for the context of emergency medical services.

The American College of Emergency Physicians (1988) published "Guidelines for Do Not Resuscitate Orders in the Prehospital Setting." This document is intended to provide procedural assistance, rather than substantive criteria for decision making.

Many administrative barriers impede the implementation of home-based "Do Not" orders. There are questions regarding the form and timeliness of documentation and procedures for authenticating orders, plus the energy needed to coordinate interacting players (e.g., patients, families, local governments sponsoring emergency squads and the agencies operating them, physicians, and home care personnel) who may be ignorant of the issues and engaged in petty but powerful turf battles (Haynes and Niemann 1985).

Fear of legal liability is a serious impediment, especially in which attorneys with no health law or bioethics background counsel as clients local municipalities who operate emergency medical squads with unreasonable, ill-informed advice to resuscitate every home care patient for whom they are called, regardless of physicians' orders to the contrary. Although special immunity statutes are not legally necessary to protect emergency medical personnel who honor a properly executed home-based DNR order, such legislation may be required psychologically to encourage desired behaviors.

In this hypothetical, where a presently incapacitated Mr. Fisher previously executed advance directives while still capable, the family's role is central in fulfilling Mr. Fisher's treatment preferences. They should support those preferences and help interpret them to members of the home care team. When decisions arise about which Mr. Fisher previously expressed no clear preference, it is up to the family (especially the daughter, who is designated the agent by the proxy directive) to guide medical conduct according to the principles of substituted judgment (i.e., what Mr. Fisher would want if presently able to make and express autonomous, authentic choices) or, if substituted judgment is not realistic, consistent with Mr. Fisher's best interests. Finally, the family needs to work with the formal home care professionals to provide informal care consistent with Mr. Fisher's wishes as long as he lives.

Case 3

In hypothetical 3, Mr. Fisher is incapable of making decisions and did not previously execute an advance directive or otherwise clearly, consistently indicate his preferences concerning life-sustaining medical interventions. Now, the role of Mr. Fisher's family would become paramount.

In most jurisdictions, Mr. Fisher's family members, in a stated priority order, would be empowered by statute to make medical decisions on behalf of their incapacitated relative with no advance instructions (Menikoff, Sachs, and Siegler 1992). The content of surrogate-decision-making statutes varies among jurisdictions, in terms of both the restrictions on the type of decision allowed and the procedural hurdles purporting to protect the vulnerable patient (Kapp 1992, 1993). Among the decisions families ordinarily are permitted to make are those pertaining to the type of prospective "Do Not" orders discussed above. Family members acting as surrogate decision makers should choose in conformity with either substituted judgment (if possible) or best-interests principles. In some states without such legislation, judicial precedent formally legitimizes the family's role.

Even without authorizing state legislation or precise judicial precedent, the longstanding medical tradition has been reliance on family members in this kind of situation (Areen 1991). This informal practice of looking to "next of kin" has been challenged only by a few commentators who want an adversary hearing and court approval for every decision to withhold or withdraw treatment for an incapacitated patient (Bopp and Avila 1991a, 1991b). The poor alternatives to reliance on next of kin, in the absence of state family consent legislation or judicial precedent legitimizing in advance the family's authority, are either routine initiation of guardianship proceedings (assuming an appropriate individual is willing and available to be named guardian by the court) or waiting until a medical emergency materializes and then intervening (e.g., by transfer to a hospital) on the basis of the emergency exception to informed consent. As a practical matter, a home health agency that is obsessed with potential liability and "that insists on a formal authorization for surrogate or substitute decision making may be unable to provide care in any fashion at all" (Dombi 1991, p. 81).

Mr. Fisher's daughter is the most appropriate surrogate decision maker (Lo, Rouse, and Dornbrand 1990) because she probably knows her father and his values best, has his best interests at heart, and will be most intimately, directly affected—as both caregiver and eventual mourner—by the decisions made and implemented. Deference to the family is not without dangers, though. In the home environment, families may find their caregiving burdens overwhelming and hence may be too anxious to bring down the final curtain. Conversely, the family that goes home after visiting a relative in a hospital or nursing home may be more willing to insist on "doing everything," since its members do not have to live quite as intensely and unrelentingly in the middle of the drama.

Professionals must be sensitive to emotional or financial conflicts of interest between the family and an incapacitated, vulnerable patient. The possibility of such a conflict, though, should not negate the usual presumption in favor of the family's acting as decisional surrogate for Mr. Fisher (Arras 1995).

Let us assume that Mr. Fisher's family, relying on a belief about what Mr. Fisher would want or an assessment of his best interests, decides to maintain Mr. Fisher at home to die without high-tech medical interventions other than palliative measures (such as patient-controlled analgesia). The family may still agree to hospitalization and treatment for intercurrent illness (e.g., broken leg) that can be reversed and whose reversal would improve Mr. Fisher's comfort and enjoyment during his remaining life. After limited treatment, he may be returned from the hospital to continue with the plan to die at home in peace.

Post-Death Issues

After Mr. Fisher dies, several things may occur that have legal and ethical ramifications. Knowing about these events might affect how the death itself is orchestrated at home.

Upon a patient's death, the attending physician usually is responsible for filling out the medical portion of the death certificate. Sometimes the attending physician is required by statute to report the circumstances of a death to a local public official, either a coroner or a medical examiner. This public official determines what steps, including an autopsy, are appropriate to investigate the death. When a case is within the coroner or medical examiner's jurisdiction, the deceased's family may not prevent a public investigation or autopsy.

State statutes differ concerning when an attending physician must report a death to the coroner or medical examiner. Standard grounds for mandatory reporting include (*a*) a reasonable belief of criminal activity, (*b*) a reasonable belief that the death was violent in nature, (*c*) the death occurred by casualty (accident), (*d*) the death was an apparent suicide, (*e*) the individual died suddenly when in apparent good health, and (*f*) the death occurred in a suspicious or unusual manner. Once a coroner or medical examiner has done an autopsy, some states treat the results as an easily accessible public document, whereas other states prevent the public from obtaining the resulting information.

These reporting and investigation requirements introduce potential retrospective oversight that may influence the willingness of physicians and other providers to implement certain treatment decisions. It may be, though, that in home care certain technological and documentation strategies are easier to employ to reduce the legal risks associated with retrospective review of potentially controversial behavior than would be the case in a health care institution.

Ideally, the agency has made prior arrangements with Mr. Fisher's physician, the local coroner, and the funeral director regarding the pronouncement of death and disposition of the body. Some families, such as those wishing to verify Alzheimer disease, might voluntarily arrange a partial or complete autopsy. The patient, while capable of making decisions, may have left permission for autopsy (e.g., for educational purposes). Acme should have written protocols detailing how these arrangements will be handled, and the specifics should be discussed ahead of time with Mr. Fisher and his family. Acme also should have a written policy on organ donation and harvesting.

Public Policy Recommendations

If home-based death is to flourish and assure dignified and autonomous final days, some of the present legal and ethical ambiguity clouding the subject must be addressed. I offer a tentative, abbreviated list of possible public policy initiatives aimed in this direction.

First, more states should consider amending their laws to permit nonphysicians to declare death under certain circumstances, such as where an expected home-based death occurs and the nurse has been certified as qualified to do this. Requiring a physician to go to the home to pronounce the obvious often results in unnecessary delay, inconvenience, and stress.

Second, an educational campaign is overdue. The public, including potential patients, families, and physicians, must be better informed about medical options at home, proper use of emergency medical systems, and surrounding ethical and legal issues (Young and Pelaez 1990). Home care professionals must be better prepared to provide timely, accurate information to those they serve (Montminy 1990).

Third, home health agencies, singly or in concert, need to develop ethics committees or equivalents to help with education, policy development and implementation, and case consultation concerning recurring ethical questions (Abel 1990). Ethics committees legitimize the importance of ethical practice, provide a conducive milieu for problem solving, and establish an intellectual framework for engaging in the decision-making process. Selling points for some form of ethics committee in home care include the changing nature of the enterprise because of technology development and concern about escalating costs, workers often acting independently without much oversight and thus getting thrust into some "tight" ethical and legal spots without sufficient support, and the lack of formal ethical preparation that most home care personnel bring to their jobs (Abel 1990, pp. 256–57).

Fourth, turf battles that inhibit the development and implementation of home-based DNR protocols that would allow panicky families to call emergency squads without subjecting the arresting patient to unwanted resuscitation attempts or other medical assaults must be worked out. Prehospital emergency providers must be educated, as must be their attorneys and the community physicians who write orders concerning the limitation of treatment for home-based patients.

Finally, society must supply more adequate resources to support families during the difficult period of caring for a dying patient at home. Home care must not mean abandoning the family. The family's tolerance for a relative dying at home depends on the support available. Can a nurse or physician come to the home to assess changes in symptoms and to help with emotional and administrative concerns at the time of death? Current organizational and financial structures frequently make this difficult (Lynn 1988). However, support needs are not always tangible. One of the reasons that families panic when even an anticipated cardiac arrest takes place is a concern with what the neighbors may think if "help" is not summoned. Home care and its emergencies do not occur in a social vacuum, and informal communities (e.g., neighbors and churches) also must be educated to support families caring for dying patients at home.

Conclusion

Dying at home is hard. It requires the support of family or other live-in companions and of physicians and other caregivers for general humanitarian and comfort care during what may be a slow and draining process. The tension between medical and social models of home care may reach a breaking point (Collopy, Dubler, and Zuckerman 1990). How we resolve and accommodate the ethical and legal questions implicated by the choice to die at home will help define home care as either just a change in the site for the provision of high-tech medical treatment or a broader change in the range of choices and services available to dying persons and in our conceptualization of care itself at the end of life.

REFERENCES

Abel, P. E. 1990. Ethics committees in home health agencies. *Public Health Nursing* 7:256–259.

American College of Emergency Physicians. 1988. Guidelines for do not resuscitate orders in the prehospital setting. *Annals of Emergency Medicine* 17:1106–8.

American Medical Association (AMA), Department of Geriatric Health. 1992. *Guidelines for Medical Management of the Home Care Patient*. Chicago: AMA.

Areen, J. 1991. Advance directives under state law and judicial decisions. *Law, Medicine & Health Care* 19:91–100.

Arras, J. D. 1995. Conflicting interests in long-term care decision making: acknowledging, dissolving, and resolving conflicts. In N. Wilson and L. McCullough, eds. *Long-Term Care Decisions: Ethical and Conceptual Dimensions.* Baltimore: Johns Hopkins University Press.

Bayer, R. 1986. Ethics in home care and quality assurance. *Caring* 5:50–56.

Bigler, B. R. 1990. Critical care nursing: Expanding roles and responsibilities within the community. *Critical Care Nursing Clinics of North America* 2:493–502.

Bopp, J., and Avila, D. 1991a. The due process right to life in Cruzan and its impact on right to die law. *University of Pittsburgh Law Review* 53: 193.

———. 1991b. Perspectives on Cruzan: The sirens' lure of invented consent: A critique of autonomy-based surrogate decisionmaking for legally incapacitated older persons. *Hastings Law Journal* 42:779–815.

Brown, L. M., and Rousseau, G. K. 1990. Resuscitation status begins at home. *American Journal of Nursing* 9:24.

Callahan, D. 1985. What do children owe elderly parents? *Hastings Center Report* 15:32–37.

Carr, P. 1992. Implications for the implementation of the Patient Self-Determination Act for nurses in the field. *Home Healthcare Nurse* 10:53–54.

Coll, P. P., and Anderson, D. 1992. Letter: Advanced directives for homebound patients. *Journal of the American Board of Family Practice* 5:359–60.

Collopy, B. 1988. Autonomy in long term care: Some crucial distinctions. *Gerontologist* 28:10–17 (suppl.).

Collopy, B., Dubler, N., and Zuckerman, C. 1990. The ethics of home care: autonomy and accommodation. *Hastings Center Report* 20:1–16 (Supplement).

Connaway, N. I. 1985. Relying on the living will in home health care. *Home Healthcare Nurse* 3:42–45.

Dombi, W. A. 1991. The patient's right of self-determination. *Caring Magazine*, May, pp. 78–82.

Dubler, N. N. 1992. *Ethics on Call: A Medical Ethicist Shows How to Take Charge of Life-and-Death Choices.* New York: Harmony Books.

———. 1990. Refusals of medical care in the home setting. *Law, Medicine and Health Care* 18:227–33.

Feinberg, E. A. 1991. Ethical issues. In M. J. Mehlman, and S. J. Youngner, eds., *Delivering High Technology Home Care*, pp. 84–124. New York: Springer.

Haddad, A. M., and Kapp, M. B. 1991. *Ethical and Legal Issues in Home Health Care.* Norwalk, Conn.: Appleton & Lange.

Havlir, D., Brown, L., and Rousseau, G. K. 1989. Do not resuscitate discussions in a hospital-based home care program. *Journal of the American Geriatrics Society* 37:52–54.

Haynes, B. E., and Niemann, J. T. 1985. Letting go: DNR orders in prehospital care. *JAMA* 254:532–33.

Johnson, S. H. 1991. Liability issues. In M. J. Mehlman, and S. J. Youngner, (eds.), *Delivering High Technology Home Care*, pp. 125–59. New York: Springer.

Joint Commission on Accreditation of Healthcare Organizations (JCAHO). 1994. *Accreditation Manual for Home Care*, vol. 1. Chicago: JCAHO.

Kapp, M. B. 1993. Restrictive state advance directive statutes: Risk management implications. *Journal of Healthcare Risk Management* 13:14–18.

———. 1992. State statutes limiting advance directives: Death warrants or life sentences? *Journal of the American Geriatrics Society* 40:722–26.

———. 1991. Health care decision making by the elderly: I get by with a little help from my family. *Gerontologist* 31:619–23.

Lo, B., Rouse, F., and Dornbrand, L. 1990. Family decision-making on trial: Who decides for incompetent patients? *New England Journal of Medicine* 322:1228–31.

Loewy, E. H. 1988. Decisions to leave home: What will the neighbors say? *Journal of the American Geriatrics Society* 36:1143–46.

Lynn, J. 1988. Commentary. In C. B. Cohen, ed., *Casebook on the Termination of Life-Sustaining Treatment and the Care of the Dying*. Bloomington, Ind.: Indiana University Press.

Markson, L., and Steel, K. 1990. Using advance directives in the home-care setting. *Generations* 14(suppl.):25–28.

Menikoff, J. A., Sachs, G. A., and Siegler, M. 1992. Beyond advance directives: Health care surrogate laws. *New England Journal of Medicine* 327:1165–69.

Montminy, A. M. 1990. Decision-making authority for family caregivers of the cognitively impaired elderly. *Journal of Community Health Nursing*, 7:215–21.

President's Commission for the Study of Ethical Problems in Medicine and Biomedical and Behavioral Research. 1983. *Deciding to Forego Life-sustaining Treatment*. Washington, D. C.: U. S. Government Printing Office.

Sachs, G. A., Miles, S. H., and Levin, R. A. 1991. Limiting resuscitation: Emerging policy in the emergency medical system. *Annals of Internal Medicine* 114:151–54.

Spiegel, A. D. 1991. Regulation of high technology home care. In M. J. Mehlman, and S. J. Youngner, eds., *Delivering High Technology Home Care*, pp. 67–83. New York: Springer.

Steel, K. 1991. Home care for the elderly: The new institution. *Archives of Internal Medicine* 151:439–42.

Thobaben, M. 1992. The legal and moral obligations of home care agencies with regard to the new Patient Self-Determination Act. *Home Healthcare Nurse* 10:55–56.

U.S. Congress, Office of Technology Assessment (OTA). 1987. *Life-Sustaining Technologies and the Elderly*. Washington, D. C.: U.S. Government Printing Office.

Young, P.A., and Pelaez, M. 1990. The in-service education program of the home health assembly of New Jersey. *Generations* 14(suppl.):37–38.

12. High-Tech Home Care in Context

ORGANIZATION, QUALITY, AND ETHICAL RAMIFICATIONS

Rosalie A. Kane, D.S.W.

This chapter examines the characteristics of home care and related quality-assurance activities in the United States. Such scrutiny is needed to draw conclusions about how high-tech home care might fit within the goals and processes of home care and to forge common understandings about standards for its quality. The aims are to explore the conditions under which high-tech home care can enhance or detract from the quality of life and the prerequisites for adequate quality. It also examines trends in the delivery of home care that might change the way all home care—including high-tech home care—is conceptualized.

The term *high tech* is imprecise, though we can recognize and agree on some of its manifestations. Typically, *high tech* includes infusion therapies (antibiotic, antiviral, pain-killing, and chemotherapy), feeding tubes (parenteral and enteral), dialysis, ventilators, and various monitoring systems (apnea monitors and cardiac monitors). This list obviously includes procedures that range widely in cost, complexity, amenability to self-administration, skill required in administration, and consequences associated with a malfunction of people or equipment. For this discussion, I take high-tech home care to refer to services that require the use of complicated equipment and materials that, if misused, could cause harm and that require special knowledge, skill, and perhaps composure to manage and monitor. The harm to the patient from a misuse of high-tech home care may come through preventable complications such as infection or injury. If the high-tech procedures or items are used to monitor an unstable condition, the harm may follow from a failure to identify detectable prob-

lems in time or at all. If the price of an error is sudden death or hor-
rendous morbidity, the stakes for this technology are obviously high.
High-tech home care is often but not always expensive, and in those
cases, questions are raised about when the care is standard for a condition as opposed to extraordinary.

High-tech care can occur almost anywhere (an electrical power
source permitting, in some cases). One must ask if it is different in
kind because it is at home. The potential dangers of high-tech care
are not, in themselves, defining. Modern medicine can cause deadly
harm even if it does not fall into the categories considered high tech
(e.g., oral drugs, catheters, wheelchairs, contact lenses); one does not
for that reason limit such items to conventional medical settings. Furthermore, the risk of physical harm is not necessarily or always
greater at home than in institutional settings. And the family members' obligations incurred by high-tech home care are also not unique.
Family members can be equally if not more firmly constrained by
their voluntary care of a family member with severe dementia as by
the care of a technology-dependent relative. It is possible, however,
that special anxieties ensue when laypersons operate complex equipment and must interpret physical reactions accurately.

To preview conclusions, this overview of home care delivery systems, financing programs, and quality-assurance strategies in the
United States leads me to the following propositions:

1. Standards for the quality of any procedure are identical, regardless of
   where the procedure is done. Arguments can be made that publicly
   financed care be delivered in the least-expensive setting. The home
   often is *more* expensive than an institution unless the patient finances
   some of the costs or receives uncompensated help from relatives or
   friends.
2. As presently organized and financed, inequities exist in who is offered high-tech care at home and in the ease of access to these services; elderly people are systematically disadvantaged.
3. High-tech home care, such as infusions, is largely being offered as a
   market "niche" service by highly specialized firms. This trend may
   have negative consequences for the overall cost and quality of home
   care.
4. In the modern era, home care has been viewed both as a substitute
   for a supposedly more expensive form of care (e.g., hospital or nursing home) and as a service with its own goals. Thus, the reimbursement of home care by public programs or private insurance is often
   conditional on its cost-effectiveness related to service or care in some
   other place. High-tech home care has often been viewed as a substitute for care in a hospital (or even an intensive care unit) and priced

accordingly, leading to high profits. Arguably, this hospital replacement is an inappropriate algorithm. In fact, some high-tech home care is almost analogous to self-care, requiring minimal professional oversight.

5. New developments in thinking about the so-called continuum of care and the place of home care within it are blurring the boundaries between home care and institutional care. New thinking about the allocation and delegation of nursing tasks may render home care less costly in relation to nursing home care. Both these features have implications for making high-tech home care more affordable and accessible.

6. Some home care programs now compensate family members under specific circumstances. These developments are likely to increase, given current directions of health care reform. It is unclear whether family members providing or assisting with high-tech care at home should be compensated, though a justification would be needed to exclude them from compensation available to those doing other forms of home care. In any event, when the so-called formal caregivers and the so-called informal caregivers occupy dual roles, quality assurance in home care will need some rethinking.

The Organization of Home Care

Historical Evolution

The roots of home care in the United States extend to nursing done in families by family members in pioneering communities, often without the benefit of formal medical advice. Depending on social status and other circumstances, the person needing care might also have been assisted by other relatives, neighbors, servants already in the household, and specially hired helpers. As the nursing profession evolved into its modern incarnation in the late nineteenth and twentieth centuries, nurses attached to public health departments, settlement houses, and emerging voluntary nursing organizations began bringing health instruction and care into the homes and apartments of urban poor people. Such nurses were agents of both their patients and the community. On the one hand, they tried to prevent or treat disease; on the other hand, acting as social agents, they tried to prevent the spread of disease. The hospital was largely a mechanism for isolating people with diseases. Until relatively recently, hospitals were dreaded places where the poor and infectious were taken against their will. Nursing homes, as we know them, were nonexistent before World War II as venues for continuing health care, though all-purpose county poorhouses lingered for centuries of American life as repositories for elderly infirm, mentally ill, and developmentally disabled persons whose kin were unable or unwilling to shelter them.

Furthermore, not too many years ago, doctors were frequently present in the homes of the sick. They had a good vantage point to recommend special-duty home "nurses" to their patients (e.g., to assist in maternal and child care after the birth of an infant, to nurse a person through a fever or a terminal illness, or to attend a household struck down with an infectious disease). Such home health workers may or may not have had formal nursing credentials.

Since World War II, medical practice has been revolutionized by potent diagnostic tools (which have rendered it impractical for physicians to do the bulk of their evaluations at home), by powerful medications, and by increasingly sophisticated surgical and medical approaches to sustaining life (which required admissions to hospitals). Activities to be undertaken by patients and their family members during a period of recuperation became more complicated. The hospital, formerly largely a place to isolate those with disease, changed character in response to the capacity to use ever more complex surgical and medical technology to cure disease and prolong life.

In the last decade or so, the pendulum has swung back to home and community care for activities formerly done in hospitals. Given greater experience with high-tech care and the miniaturization of equipment, some of the technology that fueled the growth of the modern hospital is now used in private homes and apartments. Commensurate concerns have arisen about the well-being of patients whose high-tech care is in their own hands or those of family members. Some commentators also fear for the well-being of family members, who may remain almost perpetually stressed because of the vicissitudes of administering complex regimens and procedures to very ill relatives.

The Fragmentation of Funding

In health care, form follows finance. This is particularly true of home care in the United States. This section encapsulates major funding streams for home care and resultant programs. Given the plethora of actors, the would-be overseer of quality cannot readily assign responsibility for outcomes. It is not unusual for a home care consumer, sequentially or simultaneously, to receive care from multiple paid home care providers under multiple sources of funding and to receive uncompensated care from family members and friends.

Medicare Home Health Care. Well before the enactment of Medicare, modest levels of home care for low-income families, particularly those with young children, were funded by public health dollars, and privately paying clients could purchase home care from visiting nurse agencies and privately practicing individuals. But the first big growth spurt of the home care industry followed the 1965 passage of Medicare, which provided reimbursement for home health care. Medicare beneficiaries include virtually all U.S. residents over age 65, workers certified as permanently and totally disabled, and surviving dependents of Medicare beneficiaries.

Medicare's home care benefit, as modified over the years, is highly stylized. To become a Medicare-certified home health agency, an organization must offer at least three of six specified services: skilled nursing, physical therapy, speech therapy, occupational therapy, medical social work, and home health aides. The last three services are allowable only if triggered by a need for one of the first three, and a nurse must provide supervision at intervals to the home health aide. The home health aide, moreover, was enjoined against doing any housekeeping, which would be construed as a social service.

For beneficiaries to be eligible for home health services under Medicare, they needed to have potential for rehabilitation, require intermittent care (in contrast to continuous or part-time care), and be homebound and, thus, unable to go to an outpatient setting. Initially, home health care coverage under Medicare was further circumscribed by a requirement that the beneficiary have a prior hospitalization for the specific episode of illness, though this standard was later relaxed. Through the end-stage renal disease (ESRD) program, Medicare pays for in-home renal dialysis, definitely a high-tech service. ESRD has grown rapidly since its first Medicare coverage in 1972.

In the early 1980s, Medicare began reimbursing for home hospice for those judged to be within six months of death and willing to forgo curative care. To be reimbursed as a hospice, the home health program must meet specific but rather arbitrary requirements. Although palliative rather than curative in goal, some home hospice care might be considered high tech.

Finally, in 1992 Medicare began reimbursing home health agencies for providing skilled "evaluation and management" of a case, even if no other skilled services were needed. The operational details of this provision are still being sorted out, but it seems to permit home health agencies to receive Medicare reimbursement for longer periods than previously allowed. The trade journals for home health agencies are replete with articles describing how nurses can docu-

ment the need for "evaluation and management" so that reimbursement is unlikely to be denied, as well as ways generally to maximize
Medicare reimbursement (Shuster and Clooran 1989; Stone and Krebs
1990; Johnston and Clark 1990).

As this sketch shows, Medicare-funded home care can include
high-tech components, but is not limited to them. By definition, however, Medicare funds "skilled" care that is overseen and largely delivered by professionals. Although accounting for enormous and increasingly large federal outlays, the Medicare home health care
benefit, also by definition, was insufficient to sustain a person with
long-term disability. First, the benefit was aimed at rehabilitation
rather than long-term maintenance, and it disqualified those who
were not homebound or who needed constant care. (Many people
who receive infusions and other high-tech care at home are not homebound.) Second, people needing long-term assistance often required
help with personal care and housekeeping that is labor intensive but
not highly skilled. Indeed, services such as cooking, cleaning, laundry, and shopping, which are at the opposite end of the spectrum
from high tech, are not covered under Medicare.

Thus we have a paradox. Medicare home health care is the
fastest-growing segment of Medicare. Between 1989 and 1992, its visits increased 65 percent, and the proportion of beneficiaries served
increased 63 percent. Expenditures as a total share of Medicare went
from 2.4 percent in 1988 to 5.5 percent in 1992 (Arnold, Gage, and
Harris 1994). Yet, despite this growth, the program is structured in
such a way that it is unlikely to meet the full needs of many home
care consumers.

Medicaid. Standing in contrast to Medicare-reimbursable home
care are a potpourri of more flexible programs funded by other
sources, including private pay. All states have some home care coverage under their regular Medicaid programs for low-income people
who meet the usually stringent financial eligibility requirements. Although states need not limit home care to those with rehabilitation
potential, home health care under regular Medicaid programs typically mirrors Medicare in emphasizing skilled services and thus falls
short of meeting general needs (Dombi 1991; Staebler 1991). In many
states, Medicaid also funds personal care attendant services for disabled people; these programs typically cater to people under 65,
though in some states (notably California and New York), they serve
many elderly people. States may purchase personal care from agencies or from individually employed workers, but in either case Medicaid requires that the personal care be ordered by a physician and

supervised by a nurse, and personal care workers are prohibited from doing various nursing procedures (Lewis-Idema, Falik, and Ginsburg 1991). For decades, New York, and particularly New York City, accounted for the vast majority of national home care expenditures under Medicaid.

Medicaid Waivers. In 1982, states were allowed to apply for Medicaid waivers to provide a wide array of home- and community-based services to persons with disabilities sufficient to make them eligible for nursing home care. The stipulations that can be waived include the type of service offered, Medicaid program mandates such as the requirement for state-wide uniformity, and eligibility. (Many states used waivers to expand beyond categorical eligibility for Medicaid to include people whose incomes were 200 or even 300 percent of poverty. Their aim was to serve people who, if entering nursing homes, would "spend down" to Medicaid within six months or so.) The Medicaid waiver services typically included case management, in-home services, adult day care, and home-delivered meals. All recipients had to be functionally impaired enough to be admissible to a nursing home under the state's Medicaid rules, and the program could spend on each person only a specified fraction of the average costs of nursing home care. The details of how many people could be served, the allowable services, and the per-person cap on annual expenditures are spelled out in each state's waiver applications. To be granted a waiver, the state needed to convince federal officials that the total Medicaid costs for long-term care in nursing homes and outside of nursing homes would be no greater than without it (Luehrs and Ramthun 1991). Some Medicaid waivers have been granted specifically for community care of persons with AIDS and the HIV virus (Lindsey, Jacobsen, and Pascal 1991).

To help people stay out of nursing homes, home care providers needed to meet social as well as medical needs of the clientele. Most consumers of long-term home care require regular medications, and not all can administer their own oral drugs. Some need assistance with housekeeping and transportation. Although some states opted to use home health agencies to provide home care under Medicaid waivers, others stimulated the growth of a new industry by providing payment to personal care agencies. In many states, personal care agencies are unlicensed, and typically they can provide more flexible services and charge less than do Medicare-certified agencies. In some states, most notably Oregon and Wisconsin, Medicaid waivers were used to pay independently employed workers who provide in-home services, including relatives of the person receiving care. Independently employed "personal care assistants" are more frequently reimbursed under state Medicaid programs and Medicaid waiver programs when the clientele are younger adults with disabilities.

State Programs and Aging Services Programs. Beginning in the 1970s, some states, such as Massachusetts and Pennsylvania, initiated a statewide non-means-tested home care benefit that covered the more socially oriented forms of home care, such as housekeeping, chore service, and companions. These programs have gradually expanded to cover personal care and more health-oriented services at home. Other states initiated state programs to supplement Medicaid waivers, for example, serving a group with higher incomes, lesser disabilities, or both. Typically federal block social service grants provide some funding for these efforts, though, given their failure to keep up with inflation, states often use their own general revenues as well. Until recently, one of the largest state programs was California's In-Home Supportive Services (IHSS), which in 1992 served about 170,000 clients, 55 percent of whom were over 65. Designed as a county-administered program with much local autonomy, IHSS in most counties used paid independently employed workers to give service. In 1993, this program was transferred into a regular Medicaid program, which permitted the state to receive a federal match but required adjustments to deal with Medicaid requirements for physician referral and nurse oversight.

Aging Services. Funded under Title III of the Older Americans Act, aging services are typically socially oriented services (e.g., homemaking, chore services, delivered meals, friendly visiting, and case management) provided by agencies under contract to either the state department of aging or local area agencies on aging. Although accounting for relatively few of the home care dollars, they nonetheless fill gaps in important ways. Moreover, in about one third of the states, the Older Americans Act agencies have the authority to allocate services under the Medicaid waivers. Case management is often provided directly by the area agencies on aging, which may well be responsible for waiver programs for younger adults as well as elderly people.

Insurance. Home care agencies also have a private market for their services. Individual consumers and third parties, such as insurance companies, purchase home care, often from the same home health agencies that provide it under Medicare. Some providers of high-tech home care were incorporated specifically to meet the private insurance market. Organizations that limit themselves to infusion therapy, ventilator care, and other high-tech interventions do not need to become Medicare-certified and indeed cannot become Medicare-certified unless they offer a wider range of services. Thus, those who exclusively offer infusions and similar services have opted for a lucrative "boutique" service, specializing in collecting insurance reimbursement for high-tech aspects of care that are not well covered under Medicare. Insurers tend not to balk at paying for high-tech home care because it is viewed as replacing expensive hospitals stays.

Private Pay. Home health care on a private-pay basis is unaffordable for all but the wealthy few. However, home health agencies often provide unskilled services in the home on a fee-for-service basis (e.g., aides, homemakers, and licensed practical nurses), and they may also provide private-duty nursing for time-limited periods. Some home health agencies have structured themselves with an arms-length subsidiary that does private-pay and insurance work so that they are not bound by cumbersome Medicare requirements.

Capitated programs. For members of health maintenance organizations (HMOs), home health care may well be part of the benefit package, and HMOs may use home care as a less-expensive alternative to hospitals or nursing homes. Elderly people can be members of Medicare HMOs. Such organizations receive for each elderly enrollee an annual capitated sum equivalent to the average Medicare payment in the region and, in turn, are at financial risk for providing, at a minimum, all services the older person would have received under Medicare as well as any other benefits offered in the package. Medicare HMOs may have their own home health agencies and/or contract with other providers. They have incentives to provide a wide range of hightech and low-tech home health services to the beneficiary, downshifting to less expensive forms of care. There is little evidence, however, that this is happening. In fact, recent studies (Shaughnessy and Schlenker 1993) show that Medicare HMOs provide *less* home health care to their members discharged from hospitals than the amount received by fee-for-service Medicare beneficiaries and that the former have poorer posthospital results.

The Fragmentation of Delivery Systems

The above discussion on the fragmentation of funding suggests that the provision of home care will also be a fragmented enterprise, including certified home health agencies, personal care agencies, hightech infusion agencies, and self-employed workers. But the picture is even more confusing than this thumbnail sketch would suggest, because of the myriad auspices for home care, the variation in state regulatory practices, and the propensity of home care providers to spin off subsidiary companies to respond to the different sources of funding. This, in turn, causes difficulties for those who wish to provide consumers with coherent information about how to select and evaluate home care based on quality.

Home care is presently provided by for-profit and nonprofit agencies that range in size from small organizations serving no more than a few dozen clients at any given time to multistate corporations with hundreds of thousands of clients. In terms of auspices, home care is provided by health departments (which often have been constituted as certified home health agencies), voluntary nursing associations, for-profit freestanding home care agencies, for-profit and nonprofit hospitals, HMOs, and (less often) nursing homes and public and private social service agencies. Some relationship exists between the capacity for medically oriented care, on the one hand, and size, auspice, and for-profit versus nonprofit status, on the other. For example, hospital-based programs tend to be rather small and to have the capacity for high-tech care. Social service agencies tend not to do high-tech care. For-profit home care agencies are often large. But these relationships have not been well studied, and many exceptions come to mind in the form of anecdotal data. For example, the Visiting Nurse Service in New York City, a nonprofit agency, has an unduplicated count of more than 10,000 active clients on any given day, employs a staff of more than 10,000, and can offer the full range of services from high-tech to low-tech care. Home care is also provided by independently employed workers, and in some circumstances these employees are compensated by public payor programs. Typically, low-tech services are provided under these auspices, though some registered nurses are independently employed with private-duty work. Finally, some programs also reimburse family members for providing home care (Linsk et al. 1992), though family reimbursement has largely been confined to low-tech services.

Many Medicare-certified agencies do provide high-tech services. However, specialized firms that provide only infusions and/or parenteral feedings have proliferated. Such agencies typically do not qualify to be Medicare certified because they do not offer three of the six specified services, and they largely support themselves through insurance payments. The trade literature urges Medicare-certified home health agencies to embrace high-tech home care because of both the quality-of-life improvements associated with being at home and the lucrative nature of the market (Larkins and Hellige 1992; Lindeman 1992). Moreover, the same trade literature emphasizes the need for highly skilled nursing services and large multidisciplinary teams for almost all high-tech home care, which, if accurate, would argue against specialized high-tech agencies as the optimal delivery system.

High-Tech Home Care: The Sum of Three Parts

High-tech home care is, in itself, often fragmented in funding, delivery system, or both. For much of high-tech home care, three components must come together: durable medical equipment, pharmaceuticals, and nursing services. Each has its own demands for quality assurance (Vavrinchik and Witkowski 1991; Witham-Wilson 1991). In particular, critics have lambasted the durable medical equipment industry for price excesses and lack of quality control (Mitchell 1991; Mohan and Trisler 1991; Parver 1991). Coordination of the three components of high-tech home care is not automatic. Privately insured individuals in a fee-for-service system or members of HMOs may find that all three of these components are brought together "seamlessly" and provided for by specialized infusion companies. Just as often, however, they may be forced to bring the pieces together themselves. Medicare beneficiaries may have an even more complicated task, because much high-tech home care service is not covered as part of Medicare proper.

Medicare has covered parenteral feeding for some time but does not now cover home infusions (a category that includes intravenous antibiotics, intravenous antiviral drugs, chemotherapy, and blood transfusions). Nonetheless, some Medicare beneficiaries do receive high-tech home care. Typically, these are patients whose nursing services are covered by another payor (Medicaid or Medigap insurance). Durable medical equipment is covered under Part B of Medicare. Coverage for the pharmaceuticals may also come from a non-Medicare third party or be paid for out of pocket. The U.S. Office of Technology Assessment (OTA) analyzed the implications for covering infusions under Medicare (OTA 1991). The study group judged that Medicare beneficiaries would be more likely than younger patients to need additional home health and home care services beyond the services provided by specialized infusion companies, for several reasons: their health might be more precarious; they would be more likely to live alone (thus having no family helper); and they would be more likely to have difficulties manipulating the equipment.

The options that OTA considered for adding infusions as a benefit under Medicare reveal the confusing nature of the home care marketplace. OTA considered whether the infusion benefit should be in Part A of Medicare (where most home care is located) or in Part B (where durable medical equipment is located); whether agencies certified to receive Medicare payment for infusions should be required to be multiservice agencies or whether specialized infusion agencies should be reimbursed; whether Medicare beneficiaries without family helpers should be allowed to get infusion services; and how physician services related to infusion care should be covered. Ordinarily infusion agencies pay a "consulting fee" to the referring doctor, but anti-kickback provisions of Medicare currently prohibit such payments. Physicians' services are perceived as important to the success of high-tech home care. Thus, the OTA panel tried to strike a balance between costly mandates for specified numbers of physician visits and capitated payments that might lead to underservice. The report speculated that some Medicare beneficiaries might receive care more efficiently in nursing homes or hospital swing beds but also noted that these entities have not been eager to admit elderly infusion patients.

In summary, the provisions of high-tech home care usually require juggling nursing services, durable medical equipment, and pharmaceuticals. This is not necessarily an easy task for younger home care patients and is financially prohibitive for most Medicare beneficiaries, who are currently disadvantaged for coverage of high-tech home care.

Quality Assurance in Home Care

Challenges in the Home Care Context

Quality assurance in health services is an American preoccupation, having a language and a technology all its own. Customarily, quality assurance entails a cycle of three activities: (*a*) establishing criteria or indicators of quality and setting standards; (*b*) assessing care against those criteria and standards, and (*c*) correcting problems once they are found. The criteria for quality are typically divided into structural criteria (pertaining to the program as a whole), process criteria (pertaining to the appropriateness and quality of the procedures undertaken for the particular patient), and outcome criteria (pertaining to the ultimate results) (Donabedian 1966). Standards for desired achievement are set for each criterion, on the basis of norms of professional practice, expert opinion, or research data. Care is reviewed from records, discussion with professionals, and/or direct patient assessments or interviews, usually on some sampling basis. If standards are not met, a plan of correction is introduced, which may include consultation and education, peer pressure, or punitive sanctions.

Quality-assurance activities were born in hospitals, where records are relatively detailed, professionals are dominant, and encounters with the patient are short (so that care is reviewed retroactively by reviewing the records of discharged patients). Long-term care review, in contrast, tends to include the following features: prospective review with the intent of improving the actual care of the specific person whose care is reviewed; data collection, at least in part, through direct contact with the patients; and attention to the quality of life as well as the quality of care.

Home care presents particular challenges for quality assurance. Like acute care, home care often involves specific procedures that can be reviewed for appropriateness and quality of performance. Like long-term care, home care often lasts long enough for concurrent review and correction of the care for the particular client to be possible and, therefore, morally dictated. Like ambulatory medical care, services are delivered by large numbers of people, and ultimate compliance with a regimen is up to the patient.

As suggested above, pinpointing accountability for processes and outcomes has been particularly difficult in home care. First, numerous formal agencies, independent workers, and family members simultaneously and sequentially work with the patients. High-tech home care is just an exaggerated example of that problem, because it often requires a nurse, a pharmacist, and an equipment expert for the high-tech procedure alone, but the patient may well be receiving other services at home, including domestic help and personal care. Given the multiple inputs, agencies are reluctant to take responsibility for outcomes.

Second, the home is the patient's turf, not the professional's. Home care providers cannot be expected to be in control of that environment. This shift in the balance of power in home care is in many ways a great improvement, even though nurses lament the threat to sterile procedures. On the other hand, compulsive adherence to protocols may be crucial for some high-tech procedures.

Third, family members have a particular role in relation to home care. When they are actually providing care as part of the plan, the quality of the service they offer needs to be scrutinized. Home care providers may have as a goal teaching the family how to provide care. Furthermore, family well-being is often cited as an aim of the home care enterprise, especially for so-called respite care designed to relieve family burden.

Outcomes for Home Care

Choosing the desired outcomes for home care is by no means a simple task. Different outcomes could be suggested, depending on the goal of home care (Kane et al. 1991). For example, those providing home care for the purpose of post-hospital convalescence might expect good care to result in a stabilized medical condition, patient knowledge about the health condition and its care, family knowledge about the patient's condition and care, fewer medical complications, rapid identification and treatment of any complications that arise, and fewer rehospitalizations. In addition, specific outcomes might be sought for specific health conditions.

If the goal is rehabilitation, the outcomes sought may include physical functioning and self-care ability, mobility, improved communication, and knowledge of how to compensate for disability. If the goal is to provide hospice care, outcomes examined might include pain and discomfort, patients' and families' psychological well-being, and "a good death," however that is defined and made operational. If the goal is to provide respite for family members, outcomes sought might include well-being of family caregivers, continuation of family caregivers in their supportive roles, and the client's continuation in the community.

If the home care has as its goal helping a disabled or chronically ill person live meaningfully at home, outcomes examined might include physical functioning, slowing of deterioration, consumers' satisfaction with care and perceived safety and security, timely identification of and medical attention for changes in health status, reduced nursing home admission, and, again, goals related to specific diseases and conditions. Whether the home care program should aspire to improve the psychological or social well-being of the consumers is debatable. Some would argue that home care providers should not presume that their ministrations will directly affect social factors (such as social relationships or participation) or emotional status, and they should be content that their ministrations lead to no harm in that regard. On the other hand, the home care should not be delivered in such a way that the very presence of the personnel in the home diminishes the quality of the patient's life. (Note that the term *patient* seems apt with reference to a high-tech procedure, whereas *consumer* seems to better fit an ongoing, generalized service.)

What of patient or consumer satisfaction? Surely this is a necessary measure, especially since home care providers provide intimate care in private surroundings. Yet consumers are not necessarily competent to judge technical aspects of care: a satisfied client may also be one who received care that professionals would consider below par. Outcomes can be used as indicators of quality for group information only. A single untoward outcome on many indicators does not suggest poor quality of care. Rather, outcome measures require developing an information base so that the outcomes of one care provider can be compared with those of another. Outcomes also must be adjusted for baseline status. Despite these assurances, home care providers are typically reluctant to be held accountable for outcomes, often claiming that they do not have sufficient control to be judged by the results (Kane et al. 1991). No data base is presently available about expected outcomes for patients with various characteristics who receive various kinds of high-tech home care.

Structure and Process Measures

Structural criteria of quality are the easiest to promulgate and measure. They typically refer to the qualifications of the staff, the record-keeping system, the quality of the equipment, and the various governance structures that are in place. Structural criteria have fallen somewhat into disrepute in quality assurance because they perpetuate orthodox ways of doing things and are many steps removed from outcomes. Some would argue, however, that high-tech home care requires highly qualified individuals working in teams using adequate equipment and supplies and that therefore some structural criteria are in order.

Process criteria are of two types: those related to whether a particular procedure for a particular person *should* be undertaken and those related to the adequacy of the procedure itself. The former are sometimes known as appropriateness criteria. Care is appropriate when all those who need the procedure receive it and when nobody receives it unnecessarily. Although critics often point to examples in which they believe an intervention was inappropriate (because it was futile, too expensive, or unsafe to be done at home), it is just as likely that some people lack access to appropriate high-tech home care.

Consumer and Provider Perspectives

Focus groups and survey research with consumers of home care suggest that the customers have views of their own about the quality of home care (Applebaum and Phillips 1990; Eustis, Kane, and Fischer 1993; Riley 1989). They prefer home care workers with whom they have a positive relationship, who care about them, who are compatible with them personally, who follow their instructions, who are reliable and honest, and who come and leave at the times expected.

Home care providers tend to seek process measures for quality—that is, measures that equate quality with the correct performance of care protocols. This approach lends itself particularly well to high-tech home care procedures. Protocols are available to standardize care plans (Webb and Berquist 1990), classify nursing interventions (Saba and Zuckerman 1992), and perform a wide variety of specific functions (e.g., weaning patients off ventilators at home [Glover, Bernstein, and Duffy 1992], preventing and treating skin breakdown [Harris and Peters 1990], home management of chest tubes [Garvey 1992], infusions for AIDS [Grigsby and Luque 1991], treating spinal cord injury [Hoeman and Winters 1990], or providing home dialysis [Roberts 1992]). These approaches emphasize the techniques of home care and give considerable attention to criteria for determining that a client is suitable for these procedures to be done at home.

Somehow these two perspectives—the process and structural criteria for specific procedures and the outcome measures that include consumer satisfaction—need to be brought together in considering the quality of high-tech home care. Patients cannot be expected to be able to evaluate the adequacy of the provider in the same way they might evaluate a bath or a meal. Patients need confidence in the competence of the care providers, which suggests the need for some structural criteria regarding training and some process criteria regarding procedures. But the patient's satisfaction with the care is also relevant to quality.

Quality Issues Specific to High-Tech Home Care

The notion that high-tech home care by its very nature requires especially stringent structural criteria about the training and level of personnel cries out for scrutiny. Those who take that point of view cite the harm that can occur if mistakes are made. Another, equally defensible view would match structural criteria to the competence needed to do the job rather than the harm that could ensue if it is done wrong. For example, a registered nurse's skill is not required to monitor a ventilator—families do it regularly. However, because the time is so limited for readjusting ventilator tubes that become dislodged, death can ensue if mistakes are made. Therefore, most states require shift personnel of licensed nurses to do ventilator care if no family members are available. This drives up the cost of care and reduces the volume; it also hastens the break-even point of disability, when care in an institution would be less expensive than care at home.

Home care providers are particularly conscious of liability risks in the relatively uncharted waters of high-tech home care (Johnson 1991). Most case law to date seems to concern equipment rather than nursing, but agencies are cautioned to document carefully, to seek all available accreditations, and to monitor carefully emerging federal and state standards. With these kinds of warning, it is perhaps not surprising that providers would cling to structural standards.

One unresolved structural criterion concerns the role of the physician. Representing the National Association for Home Care, geriatrician Knight Steel (1992) called for adequate reimbursement for physician presence in home care. This plea is echoed in the American Medical Association's guidelines for medical management of home care, which envisage an active, knowledgeable physician, who helps patients select a home care agency, "develops" a care plan in collaboration with others, and monitors that plan. For example, the proclaimed physician's role includes the establishment of "clear parameters for continued care, signs and symptoms to be monitored and reported, expected outcomes and potential problems" (AMA 1992, p. 12). In truth, physicians play a much more passive role, often only nominally in leadership of the effort. It is not yet clear what responsibilities should accrue to physicians for the conduct of home care and how those responsibilities should be reimbursed. On the one hand, some states have moved away from the fiction of "medical necessity" as a requirement for home care under Medicaid waivers and state programs in recognition that the service is often not truly medical. On the other hand, high-tech procedures fall under anyone's definition of "medical model." Of course, the patient will typically be under medical care for the condition requiring the high-tech home care. At issue is whether all physicians or a specialized cadre should have responsibility for monitoring care at home, and what tasks are part of the responsibility.

In the arena of high-tech home care, patient education, information, and informed consent processes would seem particularly important. One goal might be that patients themselves understand the care they are receiving well enough to provide some supervision and guidance to care providers.

Issues and Trends

Is the Medicare Beneficiary Getting a Fair Shake?

It seems indisputable that Medicare clientele are disadvantaged with regard to reimbursement for high-tech home care procedures. This situation may have arisen accidentally, and it probably continues in large part because of the high costs of covering such a large population from a public program. Some of the rhetoric on this subject seems ageist, however. Although some elderly people, like some younger people, are cognitively incapable of managing a complex regimen, many are capable of such management. The issue of covering a wide variety of high-tech procedures under Medicare brings to the surface two other issues: whether those who live alone or do not have a helping volunteer should be disqualified, and how care should be organized to provide the range of home-based services (presumed more likely to be needed by elderly clientele) in the most effective and accountable way.

Should High-Tech Specialization Be Discouraged?

Bruce Vladeck, now administrator of the Health Care Financing Administration, made the following comment in a 1993 speech: "Although touted by business analysts for their profitability, highly specialized boutique or niche agencies are real liabilities to a sustained, industry-wide effort to promote work force development, managerial sophistication and influence on the policy process" (Vladeck 1993). Vladeck was pointing to two problems with this kind of niche marketing. From a patient perspective, the quality of care may be at risk when accountability is unclear or when multiple agencies need to work with the patient. And from a system point of view, it is possible to argue that there is a social interest in prohibiting specialized, for-profit agencies to skim off the most lucrative sectors of the home care market. This weakens the ability of other agencies to provide uncompensated care.

Pricing Issues: Compared with What?

The appropriateness of high-tech home care needs to be anchored by the question "compared with what?" For example, should high-tech care be compared with forgoing care entirely? Certainly if the technology is accompanied by dubious benefits and manifest harm to the patient, forgoing it in all settings seems worth considering. Also if the technology is so expensive that it starves out other interventions for the patient (or more usually for other patients), a decision not to use it or not to "cover" its use could be entertained.

But often a high-tech procedure in home care is compared with the administration of the technology in a hospital or in a nursing home, two settings with markedly different costs. If the comparison is with keeping the patient in an institution, which would seem restrictive for the patient although perhaps cutting the family more slack, then the home care has some merit. The relative costs of care in the various settings are unfortunately hard to calculate. It is, in some ways, a product of social policy and pricing conventions both as to the profit permitted on pharmaceuticals and equipment (which should not differ by setting) and, more important, for the rules and regulations governing societal permission to administer the machines. Based on the belief that high-tech home care, in some cases, prevented hospitalization, insurance companies paid high prices for the procedures. One can ask whether this is a proper basis for setting prices when health resources are scarce. If the care can be delivered rather inexpensively at home, why should the price rise on the assumption that a hospital has been replaced? Moreover, the assumption that the patient would be in a hospital but for the home care program may be false. State Medicaid programs provide anecdotes about clients who received home care packages costing more than $200,000 a year under the authority of "hospital replacement," who later are transferred successfully to nursing homes when the home care program fails.

What if high-tech home care is compared with care in an outpatient setting, such as a physician's office? It might be proper to consider cost here, and insist that the patient go to the clinic when that is cheaper and feasible without exceeding some yet-to-be-defined harm to the patient. Some high-tech home care is a form of self-care; the patient manages the infusions or other devices with minimal monitoring from home health workers.

Blurring the Lines between Home Care and Nursing Homes

Typically home care is not cheaper than nursing home care for comparable people. Economies of scale favor the latter unless the patient needs very little, or most of what he or she needs is provided by family members. Because the unit costs for home care go down by downward substitution of personnel, mandating high-level professionals (perhaps with special additional training in high-tech procedures) to manage high-tech equipment and give high-tech care will reduce the funds available to serve more people or to provide a wider range of community services. Yet the home care journals call for more training and credentialing and for ever-larger teams.

Two trends are occurring that may work in the opposite direction, toward more parsimonious home care, including high-tech home care. First, the boundaries between home care and institutional care are breaking down (Kane 1994). Younger disabled activists are arguing that personal care should accompany them wherever they go rather than be confined to the home, and they are advocating a new, less professional model for care (Litvak, Zukas, and Heumann 1987). At the same time, new models of group residential care, known as assisted living, are offering disabled persons equivalent to those now served in nursing homes private apartments and individualized care plans. In some instances, the care is construed as home care and even delivered by home care agencies. States are struggling with how they should regulate such care and whether they should mandate that people needing high-tech procedures or people with high levels of disability be discharged to nursing homes (Kane and Wilson 1993).

The second issue is the delegation of nurse functions to less-qualified, unlicensed personnel or even to personnel with no formal health training. Family members typically provide a wide range of high-tech and low-tech services for their relatives, but when no family is available, in most states the functions revert to a nurse and quickly become more expensive than institutional care. It is not always clear whether the requirement of a nurse is based on the intrinsic skill needs—for example, to monitor a ventilator—or on the dire consequences should a mistake be made. There is a tradeoff between access to home care and the cost of individual units of service, and often there is little information about whether less-expensive personnel can do a nursing job. Risk aversion meets guild protection in a stance against delegating nursing services, but a slow trend is developing toward allowing nurses to train unlicensed personnel to do specific tasks for specific patients. If less expensive high-tech home care could be purchased, families might also be able to relieve themselves of some of their responsibilities.

Family members or the patients themselves are permitted to use virtually all home care technology (give medicines, manage catheters, preside over home dialysis, and so on). Does the danger associated with mishaps merit the insistence on nurses and supernurses around the clock if no family members are willing or able to give care? At least some states—most notably Oregon—are permitting people to receive heavy care in these homelike, normal settings. Oregon did this by modifying the nurse practice statute to allow unlicensed personnel to do any nursing function as long as a nurse has taught the person and certified his or her competence. By requiring that the teaching be both patient-specific and procedure-specific, the state believes it has built in some quality protections.

Family Compensation

There is a trend in home care to compensate family members for care when an unrelated person would also be compensated for providing the care. This is particularly true for personal care programs and low-tech programs, but there has been little discussion about compensating family members for high-tech activities. If family members are to be compensated, one needs a system to ensure the quality of the care provided by the family member. Family members should arguably meet the same quality standards as nonrelatives, especially when they are compensated for services. It will also be important to guard against pressuring patients to accept care from a family member or pressures for a family member to be the caregiver.

Concluding Comments

One can argue that if a service is indicated, it is highly likely that it can be provided at home. (If the service is futile and not worth doing, then, of course, it is not worth doing at home either.) The fragmented financing and delivery systems of home care in the United States lend themselves poorly to doing both high-tech and low-tech services at home and to pricing home care accurately. Fragmentation between sectors of care (acute hospital care, rehabilitation, primary care, home care) and the propensity to pit one against the other in terms of examining quality-cost tradeoffs also interfere with the continuity of care. Both kinds of fragmentation (within home care and between home care and other sectors of care) diminish accountability for quality. In considering the ethical issues related to high-tech home care, one should consider not only the delivery system we have now but also ways it could be changed to reduce ethical angst associated with this form of care. And in considering the quality of high-tech home care, one needs criteria related to both technical task performance and the client's satisfaction with the behavior of care providers in the client's home and their relationship with both professional and paraprofessional workers.

REFERENCES

American Medical Association (AMA). 1992. *Guidelines for the Medical Management of the Home Care Patient.* Chicago: American Medical Association.

Applebaum, R., and Phillips, P. 1990. Assuring the quality of in-home care: The "other" challenge for long-term care. *Gerontologist* 30:444–450.

Arnold, S., Gage, B., and Harris, J. 1994. *Interim Analysis of Payment Re-*

form for Home Health Services. Congressional Report C-94–02. Washington, D.C.: Prospective Payment Assessment Commission.

Dombi, W. A. 1991. Access to Medicaid home care. *Caring Magazine,* June, pp. 14–19.

Donabedian, A. 1966. Evaluating the quality of medical care. *Milbank Memorial Fund Quarterly* 4:166–206.

Eustis, N. N., Kane, R. A., and Fischer, L. R. 1993. Home care quality and the home care worker: Beyond quality assurance as usual. *Gerontologist* 33:64–73.

Garvey, C. M. 1992. A program for home management of chest tubes. *Caring Magazine,* September, pp. 78–82.

Glover, D. W., Bernstein, C., and Duffy, F. 1992. Home ventilator weaning. *Caring Magazine,* September, pp. 84–88.

Grigsby, S. F., and Luque, Y. 1991. Comprehensive, coordinated care for persons with AIDS. *Caring Magazine,* July, pp. 10–16.

Harris, M. D., and Peters, D. A. 1990. Impaired skin integrity: A nursing diagnosis—A nursing challenge. *Home Healthcare Nurse* 8:33–38.

Hoeman, S. P., and Winters, D. M. 1990. Theory-based case management: High cervical spinal cord injury. *Home Healthcare Nurse* 8:25–33.

Johnson, S. H. 1991. Liability issues. In M. J. Mehlman, and S. J. Youngner eds., *Delivering High Technology Home Care,* pp. 125–59. New York: Springer.

Johnston, J. E., and Clark, B. R. 1990. Orientation to home care: Maximizing Medicare reimbursement. *Home Healthcare Nurse* 8:45–50.

Kane, R. A. 1994. Transforming care institutions for the frail elderly: Trends in group residential care. Paper presented at Conference on Care of the Frail Elderly, sponsored by the OECD, Paris, France, 5–6 July 1994.

Kane, R. A., Illston, L. H., Eustis, N. N., and Kane, R. L. 1991. *Quality of Home Care: Concept and Measurement.* Minneapolis: University of Minnesota Long-Term Care Decisions Resource Center.

Kane, R. A., and Wilson, K. B. 1993. *Assisted Living in the United States: A New Paradigm for Residential Care for Disabled Elderly Persons?* Washington, D. C.: American Association of Retired Persons.

Larkins, F. R., and Hellige, M. 1992. Adding high-tech home care services to your agency. *Caring Magazine,* September, pp. 18–22.

Lewis-Idema, D., Falik, M., and Ginsburg, S. 1991. Medicaid personal care programs. In D. Rowland and B. Lyons, eds., *Financing Home Care: Improving Protection for Disabled Elderly People,* pp. 146–77. Baltimore: Johns Hopkins University Press.

Lindeman, C.A. 1992. Nursing and technology: Moving into the 21st century. *Caring Magazine,* September, pp. 5–10.

Lindsey, P. A., Jacobsen, P. D., and Pascal, A. H. 1991. Medicaid home and community-based waivers for acquired immunodeficiency syndrome patients. *Caring Magazine,* June, pp. 26–33.

Linsk, N. L., Keigher, S. M., Simon-Rusinowitz, L., and England,

S. E. 1992. *Wages for Caring: Compensatory Home Care of the Elderly*. New York: Praeger Press.

Litvak, S., Zukas, H., and Heumann, J. E. 1987. *Attending to America: Personal Assistance for Independent Living*. Berkeley, Calif.: World Institute of Disability.

Luehrs, J. E., and Ramthun, R. 1991. State approaches to functional assessments for home care. In D. Rowland and B. Lyons, eds., *Financing Home Care: Improving Protection for Disabled Elderly People*. Baltimore: Johns Hopkins University Press.

Mitchell, M. K. 1991. Standards for home medical equipment providers. *Caring Magazine*, November, pp. 47–49.

Mohan, K., and Trisler, P. 1991. FDA processes and practices for home use of high technology medical decision-making. In M. J. Mehlman, and S. J. Youngner, eds., *Delivering High Technology Home Care*, pp. 1915–208. New York: Springer.

Parver, C. 1991. Ethical home medical equipment business practices. *Caring Magazine*, November, pp. 40–43.

Riley, P. A. 1989. *Quality Assurance in Home Care*. Washington, D.C.: American Association of Retired Persons Public Policy Institute.

Roberts, N. H. 1992. The emancipation of at-home dialysis. *Caring Magazine*, September, pp. 30–34.

Saba, V. K., and Zuckerman, A. E. 1992. A new home health classification method. *Caring Magazine*, October, pp. 27–34.

Shaughnessy, P. W., and Schlenker, R. 1993. *Cost-Effectiveness of Home Health Care Under Fee-for-Service and Capitated Payment*. Colorado Springs: University of Colorado Center for Health Services Research, mimeo.

Shuster, G. F., and Clooran, P. 1989. Nursing activities and reimbursement in clinical case management. *Home Healthcare Nurse* 7:10–15.

Staebler, R. 1991. Medicaid providing health care to (some of) America's poor. *Caring Magazine*, June, pp. 4–14.

Steel, K. 1992. Homeward bound. *Caring Magazine*, October, pp. 9–12.

Stone, C. L., and Krebs, K. 1990. The use of utilization review nurses to decrease reimbursement denials. *Home Healthcare Nurse* 8:13–18.

U.S. Congress, Office of Technology Assessment (OTA). 1991. *Home Drug Infusion Therapy under Medicare*. OTA-H-510. Washington, D.C.: OTA.

Vavrinchik, D., and Witkowski, A. 1991. Standards and accreditation for durable medical equipment providers. *Caring Magazine*, November, pp. 44–46.

Vladeck, B. 1993. Home-based care for a new century. Speech given at meeting sponsored by the Milbank Memorial Fund and the Visiting Nurse Service of New York City, Harriman, N.Y., 8 November 1993.

Webb, L. A., and Berquist, S. L. 1990. Standardized care plans for home care. *Home Healthcare Nurse* 8:21–29.

Witham-Wilson, M. 1991. A survey of home respiratory equipment suppliers' practices. *Caring Magazine*, November. pp. 50–74.

13. The Economic Impact of High-Tech Home Care

*Peter S. Arno, Ph.D., Karen Bonuck, Ph.D.,
and Robert Padgug, Ph.D.*

The resurgence of home medical care as an alternative to hospitalization is in a sense a return to the past. Before World War II, the dearth
of institutional facilities meant that treatment and care had to be delivered at home. When the war ended, technologically advanced hospitals were built on a large scale and quickly became the "modern"
and preferred way to deliver care.

Over the past twenty years, the pendulum has swung dramatically in the opposite direction, and an increasing share of the nation's
health care dollar has been apportioned to home care. In 1970, expenditures for hospital care exceeded those for home care by a margin of
279 to 1; by 1991, this margin had shrunk to 29 to 1 (Letsch 1993).
Another recent shift came as high-tech home care began to play a
more prominent role in the home care market, beginning in the early
1980s. It has increasingly become an alternative to hospitalized care
rather than just a means of recovering from it.

This chapter uses an economic perspective to examine high-tech
home care and the industry that provides it. In the first section, we
define high-tech home care and describe its major cost components.
The second section charts the growth of high-tech home care, identi-
fies the factors that promote its use, and examines economic costs
and reimbursement mechanisms, particularly as they relate to the
claim that high-tech home care saves money. In the third section, we
discuss industry pricing practices and the problems associated with
the absence of regulation. This chapter draws heavily on examples
from the treatment of people with the human immunodeficiency virus (HIV), which has fueled much of the industry's recent growth.

Background: What Is High-Tech Home Care?

While traditional home care focuses on the provision of personal care and housekeeping assistance, high-tech home care involves the use of more sophisticated apparatus, such as infusion therapy to provide nutrition or medication, medical devices to monitor the patient, and ventilator systems that provide assistance with breathing. We concentrate here on infusion therapies, which have expanded rapidly, are extremely costly, and are increasingly used in the treatment of HIV and cancer.

Under some circumstances, infusion therapy must be administered by skilled nurses, but technological refinements have made it easier for family members or other caregivers to provide most necessary patient care, and treatments can even be administered by patients themselves in some circumstances. Infusion therapy delivers nutrients or medications, requires specialized equipment and infusion solutions, and can be administered by two different routes. Enteral feeding, sometimes referred to as tube feeding, is used to infuse nutrients and water into the stomach or intestine when the gastrointestinal tract is unable to digest and absorb food normally. Parenteral feeding (also known as total parenteral nutrition, or TPN) infuses nutrients and water into the veins through a catheter, bypassing the gastrointestinal tract (OTA 1987).

There are many nutritional applications of home infusion therapy for persons with HIV. For example, they are used to provide fluids to counter the severe dehydration that accompanies opportunistic infections and to treat the weight loss that characterizes generalized wasting syndrome (Mello-Udine 1992).

Home antibiotic therapy to treat infections has historically been administered intravenously through drip flow systems. However, more sophisticated infusion devices allow greater control over the flow of drugs and, as a result, permit the use of more complex medications. For example, HIV-infected patients now receive Bactrim or pentamidine for the treatment and prevention of *Pneumocystis carinii* pneumonia and ganciclovir and foscarnet to treat cytomegalovirus and herpes infections (Mello-Udine 1992).

The direct costs of high-tech home care are primarily for medications, equipment and supplies, and personnel. Indirect costs include program administration, training, and marketing.

—*Medications.*   A direct cost of high-tech home care is the medication or nutritional supplement. In theory, the unit cost per dose should be the

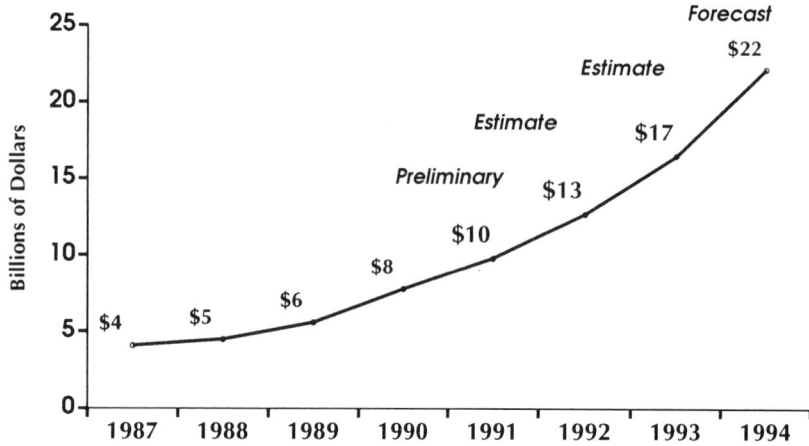

Figure 13.1.   U.S. home care expenditures (in billions of dollars). *Source:* Data from U.S. Department of Commerce, 1994

same in inpatient and outpatient settings. However, home care agencies often include a preparation or admixing fee in the cost of solutions, partly to cover personnel and administrative costs. If patients are permitted to mix their own solutions, costs may be reduced (Brakebill et al. 1983). In general, these drug costs are rising because the newer antibiotic infusion therapies, such as ganciclovir or foscarnet, tend to be considerably more expensive than standard antibiotics, such as penicillin.

—*Medical equipment and supplies.*   Equipment costs depend on the route of administration. Infusion pumps are typically more costly than the older drip flow antibiotic systems (New et al. 1991).

—*Personnel.*   The wages, benefits, and fees involved in a high-tech home care program typically include direct patient care, telephone consultation, and patient monitoring by nurses and physicians. Where family members or other caregivers are able to administer these therapies, the associated costs may be reduced.

Industry Growth

The home care industry has ballooned in the past decade. In 1987, $4 billion was spent on home care in the United States; by 1994, the figure was expected to grow to $22 billion (fig. 13.1). The home infusion therapy market alone grew from less than $1 billion in 1987 to $3.3 billion in 1993 (fig. 13.2).

At least a portion of the rise in home health expenditures (particularly the high-tech portion) is directly attributable to AIDS. The costs of outpatient care as a percentage of the lifetime costs of treating

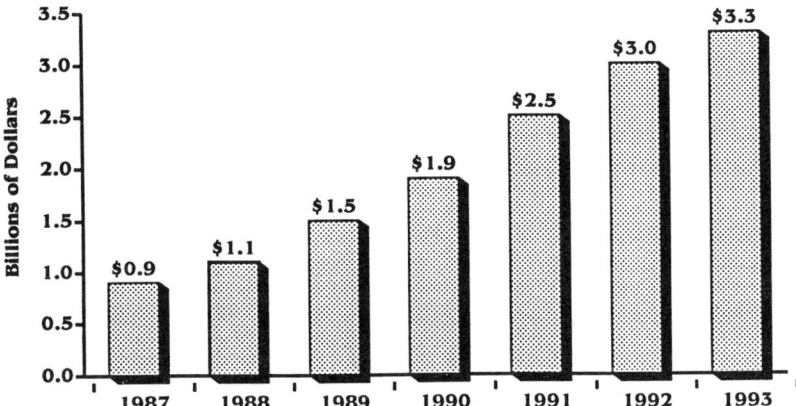

Figure 13.2. The U.S. home infusion therapy market, 1987–1993. *Source:* Data from Generio T. Gargiulo, Executive Vice-President, Barington Capital Group, L.P., 1994

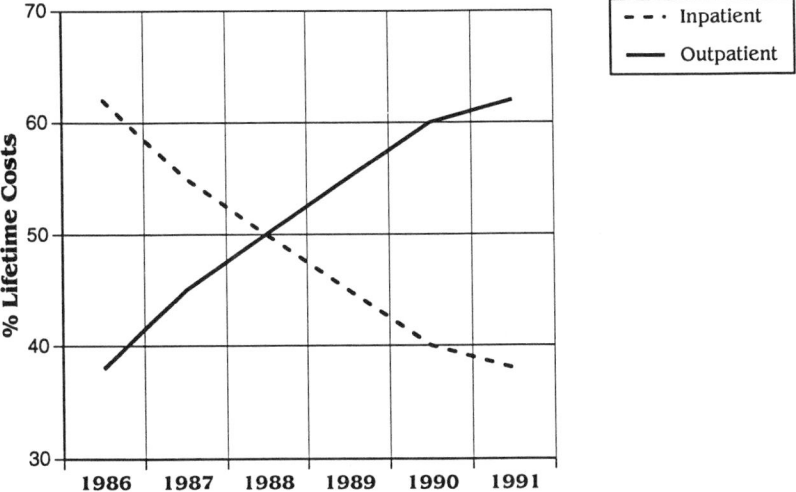

Figure 13.3. AIDS inpatient versus outpatient lifetime treatment costs, 1986–1991. *Source:* Data from Empire Blue Cross and Blue Shield

AIDS have grown while the costs of inpatient care have declined proportionately. In 1991, at Empire Blue Cross and Blue Shield, the country's largest private insurer of persons with HIV infection and AIDS, more than 60 percent of the total costs for an average AIDS patient with both hospital and major medical insurance was for outpatient services, compared with less than 40 percent in 1986 (fig. 13.3). TPN

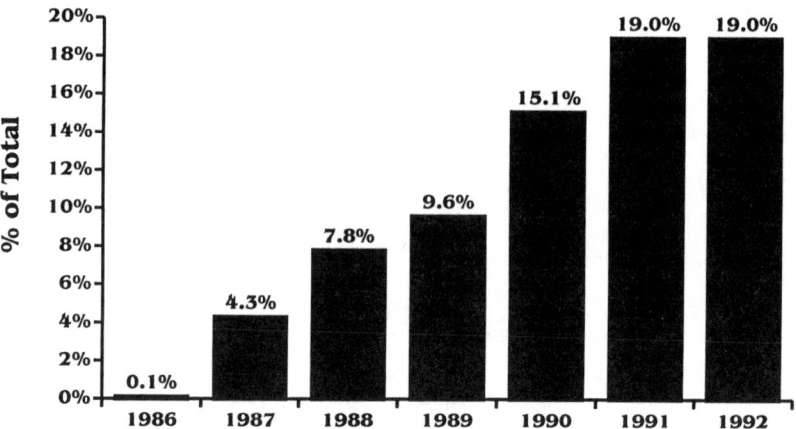

Figure 13.4.   Total parenteral nutrition as a percentage of all AIDS-related major medical payments. *Source:* Data from Empire Blue Cross and Blue Shield

is one of the major factors driving up AIDS-related costs. TPN as a proportion of all of Empire's AIDS-related major medical payments (exclusive of inpatient care) increased from less than 1 percent in 1986 to 19 percent in 1992 (fig. 13.4).

The Appeal of Home Care

While the effort to contain costs is an important factor explaining the growth in high-tech home care (discussed in greater detail below), patient preferences, technological advances, and the availability of third-party financing have also had a significant impact. Home care has had special appeal among the AIDS population, which is relatively young, because it offers more autonomy and independence (Carney 1990). The demand for greater patient involvement in treatment, which was spawned in part by the AIDS epidemic, has also enhanced the attractiveness of high-tech home care.

Refinement in the medical equipment used to deliver therapies is another factor central to the growth of the high-tech home care industry. A number of biotechnology drugs, including colony-stimulating factors to treat cancer and AIDS, as well as other AIDS drugs discussed earlier, are efficiently delivered through infusion. Current devices more precisely regulate the rate of infusion, allowing nutrients and medications to be administered at specified dosages and on a routine schedule.

A third element in the growth of high-tech home care is expanded insurance coverage. Private-sector insurers provide the bulk of revenues for infusion therapy, although policies vary, and few studies have described the extent and breadth of available coverage. One assessment is that private insurance plans usually pay 80 to 90 percent of the cost of infusion drug therapy; the remaining costs are charged to the patient (Giglione 1988), although infusion companies are often reported to waive patient copayment requirements to attract and retain individual customers.

Medicare began to cover limited aspects of home parenteral and enteral nutrition in the mid-1970s (OTA 1992). However, there is no comprehensive home drug-infusion benefit per se under Medicare. Coverage is administratively fragmented between Medicare Parts A and B, and the particulars of what are covered vary from one carrier to another.

Federal law does not explicitly define home health services under the Medicaid program, and coverage varies by state, but nearly all programs provide home care services under Section 2176 waivers. Waivers, granted by the federal government, allow states to offer a Medicaid benefit to certain people under specified circumstances, in effect waiving some state requirements that would otherwise be in effect. Federal legislation allows areas with operating Section 2176 waivers to use Medicaid funds to provide home care services for people who would otherwise require institutional care, as long as the waiver services are less costly. As a result, Medicaid is typically more liberal in its coverage of high-tech home care than Medicare and even some private insurance plans. About one-third of states have home- and community-based waivers targeted specifically for persons with AIDS.

Third-party reimbursement to individuals is just one piece of the financial pie promoting the use of high-tech home care. Shifts in the way hospitals are reimbursed have also been a boon to the industry. With the widespread adoption of prospective reimbursement in the 1980s, hospitals were rewarded financially for reducing lengths of stays. To the extent that high-tech home care was perceived as shortening inpatient stays, its growth was supported by hospitals. The doubling of home health expenditures between 1987 and 1990, the years after the prospective payment system was implemented, tends to support this contention.

Cost Containment: Is It Real?

Perhaps the most important factor fueling the growth of the high-tech home care industry is the struggle to contain health care costs. Beginning in the late 1970s and continuing through the mid-1980s, a spate of studies compared the costs of administering antibiotic and nutritional therapy at home with comparable hospital treatment and concluded that high-tech home care was more cost-effective for similar patients with similar conditions. For example, a twenty-person study of home parenteral antibiotic therapy found that average daily inpatient charges were four times higher than outpatient charges (Antonislis et al. 1978). Other researchers found that administering parenteral antibiotics at home for bone and tissue disorders saved $5,728 over hospital treatment (Rehm and Weinstein 1983). Similar claims of cost savings from home infusion therapy are found throughout the literature (Balinsky and Nesbitt 1989; Chamberlain et al. 1988; Grizzard, Haris, and Karns 1991; Kind, Williams, and Gibson 1985; Spiegel 1991a, 1991b; Stiver et al. 1978). A comparison of charges for parenteral nutrition programs found that hospital charges were four times higher than charges at home, although excluding the cost of the bed rendered the two almost equal (Brakebill et al. 1983). Similar findings from other home parenteral nutrition programs have been reported (Detsky et al. 1986; Dzierba et al. 1984).

A number of caveats to these findings are warranted. First, most studies addressed the use of parenteral or enteral antibiotic therapies, which have traditionally been less expensive than nutrition therapies. Second, hospitalized patients may differ, either clinically or in other ways, from patients maintained at home. Specifically, the study populations treated at home tended to have fewer complications and had support systems to help prepare and administer the infusion. Similarly, some studies compare home care costs with actuarially (expected) based lengths of hospital stays, despite the fact that some patients are in fact discharged earlier. In addition, some of the data sources used to conclude that home care saves money may be inconsistent. For example, Eisenberg and Kitz (1986) found enormous variations in the estimated savings from outpatient antibiotic therapy when different sources of data for hospital costs were used. It is certainly possible that the total costs associated with high-tech home care, including equipment, drugs, and possibly round-the-clock nursing, can in certain circumstances be more expensive than hospital treatment. This has certainly been the experience of Empire Blue Cross and Blue Shield in New York City, for example, and anecdotal evidence suggests that it is common elsewhere as well. Whether costs will be higher or lower depends on many factors, including the intensity of the care required by individual patients, the amount of nursing and other services they need, and the type of reimbursement system in place; in areas in which DRG systems have been implemented for inpatient reimbursement, for example, hospitalization may well produce better results (from the cost point of view, at least).

The shift to home care may also contain some hidden costs to the hospital. If the beds vacated by patients suitable for home care are filled by more resource-intensive or long-staying patients, the hospital may not be fully reimbursed for its services. Alternatively, if these beds are left vacant, hospitals may lose revenues or seek to shift costs to the remaining patients and their insurers through surcharges and rate increases (Freudenheim 1992).

Finally, cost-effectiveness is generally analyzed from the perspective of the hospital or insurer. When a broad social perspective is considered, additional costs may be taken into account. For example, the costs to a household of managing a patient receiving high-tech services at home may include the lost earning power of home caregivers and the cost of retraining workers who leave their jobs to assume these roles, the emotional cost to household members of caring for the patient, and the loss of family mobility.

Apart from costs, the circumstances under which persons are discharged from a hospital to high-tech home care must be considered. Especially among persons without adequate social supports or an appropriate home environment, the move to high-tech home care can be a disservice. For instance, nutritional therapies are now routinely administered to persons with AIDS living in single room occupancies and welfare hotels. The absence of hygienic conditions and support services in such environments may make home-based infusion therapy unsafe.

Today's doubts about the true value of high-tech home care parallel the finding over the last decade that community-based care was not a panacea for rising hospital costs. In fact, the most comprehensive evaluations found that community care rarely reduced the use of outpatient or inpatient services and that overall health care costs often increased. In addition, although patients reportedly felt better being cared for in the community, the physical benefits of community care were hard to prove (Weissert 1985).

More research is needed to make a meaningful assessment of cost-effectiveness and the relative well-being of patients who are hospitalized and those who are receiving high-tech home care. One of the few longitudinal studies conducted in this area involved 1,594 patients in seven disease categories who received home parenteral nutrition (Howard et al. 1991). Researchers concluded that the quality of clinical outcomes justified such therapy for many people with serious, long-term chronic illness, but they questioned its utility and appropriateness in some cases of end-stage cancer or AIDS, where expected survival was relatively short and additional therapy was unlikely to change the outcome. Overall, there is a lack of convincing scientific evidence to suggest precisely when high-tech home care is either medically appropriate or cost-effective.

Another serious problem involves the quality of high-tech home care in general. Nationally recognized standards for high-tech home care providers have been relatively late in coming, and not all home care companies apparently follow even those that exist (Feinberg 1991; Margolis 1993; Spiegel 1991a). State regulations, as in other areas, vary considerably, while federal regulation is largely absent.

The Price of High-Tech Home Care: Fair or Fudged?

Between 1987 and 1994, the average annual increase in home care expenditures was 27.5 percent, compared with an average annual rise of 11.5 percent for overall national health expenditures (fig. 13.5). This rate of increase outstripped every other service sector of the health care industry, including hospital care, physician services, nursing home care, and administrative costs.

In addition to the increased utilization of high-tech home care by greater numbers of people, rising expenditures in this sector reflect, in part, the industry's pricing practices. Variations in charges are endemic. In a 1990 study, the U.S. General Accounting Office (GAO) examined the fees charged by 57 Medicare carriers for durable medical equipment, such as ventilator systems, used at home. The GAO found that fees varied by 100 percent for 95 percent of the items surveyed; for more than 40 percent of those, there was as much as a sixfold difference in prices (GAO 1990). In another study, the federal Health Care Financing Administration (HCFA) discovered similar discrepancies and reported "very wide variance in charges among home intravenous drug therapy providers for comparable service" (*Medicare* 1989). An investigation by New York City's Department of Consumer Affairs also identified price differences of more than 100 percent charged by high-tech home care providers in New York City (City of New York DCA 1991).

Another pricing issue is the huge disparity between costs to the company and charges to the consumer. The HCFA study, for example, noted a weak relationship between costs and charges. Table 13.1 illustrates the structure of the TPN market, which allows a company to bill $15,000 a month for supplies and solutions that actually cost $2,200. These markups lend credibility to the contention that the

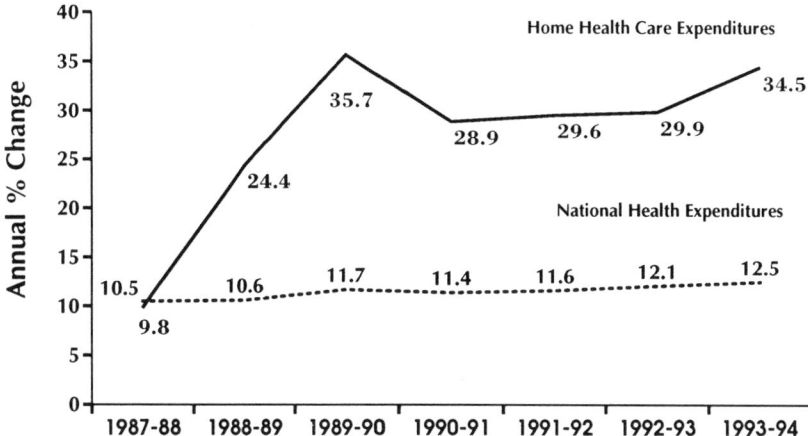

Figure 13.5.   U.S. home care versus national health expenditures, annual percentage change. *Source:* Data from U.S. Department of Commerce, 1994

high-tech home care industry is making large profits at the expense of patients and insurance companies and may be eliminating the cost advantage of providing care at home (*AIDS* 1990). However, because the industry is largely unregulated, neither public nor private payers have been able to obtain the data necessary to pinpoint more precisely the relationship between costs and charges.

The absence of regulation also allows the high-tech home care industry to bundle services, negotiate prices with insurers, and engage in bidding practices without informing other purchasers (Curtiss 1988). Additionally, some home health agencies and suppliers have

Table 13.1.
The home infusion therapy market: (typical?) example of costs and markups[a]

Item	Monthly Usage	Approximate Cost ($)	Billing Rate ($)
TPN solution (pharmacy fee included)	30	2,293	9,000
Intralipids/half liter (fatty supplements)	12	224	1,489
Administration kit (gauze, syringe, etc.)	30	476	2,877
Central line supply kit (catheter and supplies)	12	138	923
Intravenous pump rental	30 days	64	675
Pole rental	30 days	6	50
Total		2,201	15,014
Gross profit		12,813	

Source: Business Week, 11 June 1990, with permission.
[a]Prescription: 2 liters a day for a month of total parenteral nutrition therapy (a solution of amino acids, dextrose, and fatty supplements fed intravenously)

been able to screen for more profitable patients by carefully monitoring their patient and payer mix. The New York City Department of
Consumer Affairs investigation indicated that individuals with private insurance are generally served by for-profit home care agencies.
By contrast, Medicaid clients and individuals with inadequate insurance, who typically have the most severe medical or social service
needs, are more likely to receive care from the not-for-profit agencies
such as the Visiting Nurse Service (City of New York DCA 1991).

The ability of the industry to set its own prices—and largely on
its own terms—appears to be coming to an end as private-sector insurers have begun to take steps to lessen their liability and to exercise
greater leverage over the reimbursement for TPN and other high-tech
home care services. Since these services were developed relatively
recently and their costs, until the last few years, represented only a
small proportion of total costs for any particular payer, they tended
to escape the close scrutiny that other health services, particularly
inpatient hospital services, began to receive in the 1980s. But as both
the utilization and the costs of these services have rapidly increased,
and as private insurers have become increasingly more interested in
managing the costs of chronic illness in general and of AIDS in particular, they have begun to demand greater accountability on the part
of high-tech care companies, more reliable cost data from them, and
a more favorable pricing structure (Jones 1992).

Many insurers are demanding, and receiving, discounts from
high-tech home care company charges of as much as 60 percent (Cohen and Dorfman 1992). Empire Blue Cross and Blue Shield, for example, has created a home infusion network that includes a small
number of companies willing and able to provide such discounts, and
other Blue Cross and Blue Shield companies have done the same (Anders 1993; Freudenheim 1992).

It is significant in this respect, for example, that a bill before the
last Congress (H.R. 4128 and S. 1967) would have, among other
things, forced providers to be licensed by the state in which they are
headquartered, banned physician referrals to infusion companies in
which physicians have a financial stake, and mandated that the Department of Health and Human Services create uniform payment
rates for infusion services.

Pressures from payers and the increasing scrutiny of both the
pricing policies of, and the quality of care delivered by, high-tech
home health companies are beginning to have major effects on the
industry as a whole. During the heady years of the 1980s, when entry
into the high-tech market was relatively easy and profits were tempt-

ingly large, the industry was overrun by a large number of relatively small companies, often owned directly by pharmacies or physicians, with narrow market niches and relatively restricted service capacity (Jones 1985; OTA 1992; Speigel 1991b). As prices have been forced down by third-party payers and as greater scrutiny of capacity and quality has begun to have some impact, many of these small "players" have been forced out of the market or have been bought up by larger companies with greater financial and servicing capacity (*Home Care* 1994). Anecdotal evidence increasingly suggests that many smaller companies, unable to expand beyond the home infusion market and incapable of lowering their costs sufficiently, have even begun to operate at a loss and will eventually be forced to leave the market. As a result of these trends, the most forward-looking and flexible companies, such as Caremark, are rapidly diversifying into pharmaceuticals, physician practice management, and related areas, as well as seeking a more important role in the growing market for case management services for AIDS and other chronic and expensive diseases.

Conclusion

The use of sophisticated technologies to provide nutritional and antibiotic therapies at home has grown tremendously during the past ten years. Like many innovations, high-tech home care was eagerly embraced by patients and health care providers as a lower-cost, more patient-centered approach to treatment. The availability of reimbursement through public and private insurance programs improved its access to patients. Likewise, hospitals perceived home care as a way to discharge patients earlier and therefore to prosper under the new prospective payment system. Together, these factors fueled the swift growth of what appears to be an extremely profitable industry.

However, high-tech home care has not proven to be the panacea that it was expected to be, at least partly because oversight has been largely absent. Despite claims to the contrary, the cost-effectiveness of home care is called into question by high prices that often bear little relationship to costs. The absence of research to determine when high-tech home care is clinically appropriate raises doubts about its widespread use. While there may, in fact, be significant advantages over similar, hospital-delivered care, more information is needed before high-tech home care can assume an unquestioned role in the continuum of health care.

The high-tech home care industry is clearly undergoing major changes at present. Precisely what it will look like in the future is uncertain—a small number of relatively large firms is likely to dominate it completely—but it is certain that it will have to conform to the increasingly competitive and cost-conscious standards now being imposed on the rest of the health care world or it may not be able to survive at all.

REFERENCES

AIDS home care may be due for some housecleaning. 1990. *Business Week*, 11 June, p. 20.

Anders, G. 1993. Massachusetts Blue Cross's expected cut in infusion costs shows insurers' clout. *Wall Street Journal*, 2 November, p. A4.

Antonislis, A., Andersen, B. C., Van Volkinburg, E. J. V., Jackson, J. M., and Gilbert, D. N. 1978. Feasibility of outpatient self-administration of parenteral antibiotics. *Western Journal of Medicine* 128:203–6.

Balinsky, W., and Nesbitt S. 1989. Cost-effectiveness of outpatient parenteral antibiotics: a review of the literature. *American Journal of Medicine* 87:301–5.

Brakebill, J. I., Robb R. A., Ivey M. F., Christensen D. B., Young J. H., et al. 1983. Pharmacy department costs and patient charges associated with a home parenteral nutrition program. *American Journal of Hospital Pharmacy* 40:260–63.

Carney, K. L. 1990. AIDS care comes home: Balancing benefits and difficulties. *Home Healthcare Nurse* 8:32–37.

Chamberlain, T. M., Lehman, M. E., Groh, M. J., Munroe, W. P., and Reinders, T. P. 1988. Cost analysis of a home intravenous antibiotic program. *American Journal of Hospital Pharmacy* 45:2341–45.

City of New York, Department of Consumer Affairs (DCA). 1991. *Making a Killing on AIDS: Home Health Care and Pentamidine*, May.

Cohen, L. P., and Dorfman, J. R. 1992. Home infusion care providers face pressure on stock prices from cost-conscious insurers. *Wall Street Journal*, 8 June, p. C2.

Curtiss, F. R. 1988. Recent developments in federal reimbursement for home health-care services and products. *American Journal of Hospital Pharmacy* 45:1682–90.

Detsky, A. S., McLaughlin, J. R., Abrams, H. B., et al. 1986. A cost-utility analysis of the home parenteral nutrition program at Toronto General Hospital. *Journal of Parenteral and Enteral Nutrition* 10:49–57.

Dzierba, S. H., Mirtallo, J. M., Grauer, D. W., et al. 1984. Fiscal and clinical evaluation of home parenteral nutrition. *American Journal of Hospital Pharmacy* 41:285–91.

Eisenberg, J. M., and Kitz, D. S. 1986. Savings from outpatient antibiotic therapy for osteomyelitis. *JAMA* 255:1584–88.

Feinberg, E. A. 1991. Ethical issues. In M. J. Mehlman and S. J. Youngner, eds., *Delivering High Technology Home Care*, pp. 81–124. New York: Springer.

Freudenheim, M. 1992. A squeeze hurts a health niche, *New York Times*, 2 September, p. D2.

Giglione, L. 1988. Home IV therapy: Who pays? *Journal of Intravenous Nursing* 11:294–96.

Grizzard, M. B., Haris, G., and Karns, H. 1991. Use of outpatient parenteral antibiotic therapy in a health maintenance organization. *Review of Infectious Diseases* 13:S174-S179.

Home care consolidations seen aiding network contracting. 1994. *PPO Letter* 4:1,3.

Howard, L., Heaphey, L., Felming, R., Lininger, L., and Steiger, E. 1991. Four years of North American registry home parenteral nutrition outcome data and their implications for patient management. *Journal of Parenteral and Enteral Nutrition* 15:384- 393.

Jones, D. C. 1992. Electronic network could cut costs of homecare, *National Underwriter*, 1 June, 18.

Jones, G. 1985. The best-kept secret in home health care. *Rx HomeCare* 7:9.

Kind, A. C., Williams, D. N., and Gibson, J. 1985. Outpatient intravenous antibiotic therapy. *IV Antibiotic Therapy* 77:105–1.

Letsch, S. W. 1993. National health care spending in 1991. *Health Affairs* 12:94–110.

Margolis, R. E. 1993. The home infusion industry: Patients' angel or their ruthless plunderer. *HealthSpan* 10:18–20.

Medicare program; payment for home intravenous drug therapy services. 1989. *Federal Register*, 11 November.

Mello-Udine, L. 1992. Home care for AIDS patients. *New Jersey Medicine* 89:52–54.

New, P. B., Swanson, G. F., Bulich, R. G., and Taplin, G. C. 1991. Ambulatory antibiotic infusion devices: Extending the spectrum of outpatient therapies. *American Journal of Medicine* 91:455–60.

Rehm, S., and Weinstein, A. J. 1983. Home intravenous antibiotic therapy: A team approach. *Annals of Internal Medicine* 99:388–92.

Spiegel, A. D. 1991a. Regulation of high technology home care. In M. J. Mehlman and S.J. Youngner, eds., *Delivering High Technology Home Care*, pp. 67–83. New York: Springer.

———. 1991b. The economics of high technology home care: Doing right for the wrong reason. In M. J. Mehlman and S. J. Youngner, eds., *Delivering High Technology Home Care*, pp. 23–66. New York: Springer.

Stiver, H. G., Telford, G. O., Mossey, J. M., et al. 1978. Intravenous antibiotic therapy at home. *Annals of Internal Medicine* 89:690–93.

U.S. Congress, Office of Technology Assessment (OTA). 1987. *Life-sustaining Technologies and the Elderly*. Washington, D.C.: Government Printing Office.

——. 1992. *Home Drug Infusion Therapy under Medicare*. Washington, D.C.: Government Printing Office.

U.S. General Accounting Office (GAO). 1990. Medicare: Durable medical equipment fee schedules have widely varying rates. Statement of Janet Shikles, Director of Health Financing and Policy Issues. House of Representatives Subcommittee on Ways and Means, 2 May.

Weissert, W. G. 1985. Seven reasons why it is so difficult to make community based long term care cost effective. *Health Services Research* 20: 423–33.

14. Justice and Access to High-Tech Home Care

Norman Daniels, Ph.D.

Two Questions of Fairness

Home health care, and especially high-tech home care, is the fastest-growing area in health care services. For example, the home infusion market for AIDS alone reached $575 million in 1991 (City of New York DCA 1991, p. 6); with the continued growth of the HIV-infected population, this market will expand significantly in the next decade. Other high-tech home services enjoying spectacular growth include new ventilator and monitoring technologies.

Two forces propel the growth of home health care, one on the demand side, the other shaping supply (Mehlman and Youngner 1991). First, many people would rather remain among their family and friends for care than in hospitals. Indeed, for many AIDS patients with compromised immune systems, hospitals can be dangerous places. More than that, the increasing demand for home health care is a result of other partial successes in our health care system. People with HIV infection live longer: this is the much-heralded conversion of an acute disease into a chronic one. The effect, however, is that they must be treated more intensively and more expensively. Neonates who would have died years ago are now treated aggressively, but a large proportion of those who survive are disabled and need long-term intensive treatment. The rapid growth of the "old-old," a trend projected to last well into the next century, assures a growing demand for these technologies and services.

The second force consists of measures aimed at cost containment

An earlier version of this chapter appeared in *Seeking Fair Treatment: From the AIDS Epidemic to National Healthcare Reform* by Norman Daniels, © 1995 Oxford University Press.

and cost shifting. These measures shape or direct the supply of resources away from institutional services and toward home health services. Hospitals are very expensive hotels. Moving even quite ill but relatively stable patients out of hospitals and into their homes can yield great savings, especially for third-party payers. Of course, there is some inevitable cost shifting here: home expenses rise. Families and friends contribute labor time, even when there is also nursing care, often at the expense of earnings. These costs do not show up on the ledgers of public or private third-party payers, and from a societal point of view, they constitute cost shifting rather than true cost savings. Furthermore, we do not have good information about how much of the provision of high-tech home care is a substitute for hospital-based technology and how much constitutes additional services that might have been foregone had they not been available in the home.

These demand and supply forces not only have produced the recent rapid growth of high-tech home care but also threaten to continue unabated. As a result, we see huge quantities of health care resources drawn into a new area of expenditure at just the time that we are becoming most aware that we cannot provide all "medically necessary" or medically beneficial services and that we must develop new ways of limiting or rationing care. Moreover, many of these services are aimed at people who have irreversibly compromised quality of life and may be dying. For some commentators, like Callahan (1987), who have urged that we substitute "high touch" care for "high tech" care for those who are very near the end of life or for whom we can do little, the burgeoning high-tech home care industry looms as a perversion of their goal. They press the questions, Should we be developing these technologies on this scale? Aren't there better things we could do with our scarce medical resources? By expending resources on these new technologies, aren't we being unfair to others with more important needs elsewhere in the health care system or even elsewhere in society (e.g., the educationally underserved)? Ironically, reimbursements have flowed toward high-tech home care in part to save resources, but shouldn't we bite the bullet harder and simply turn off the spigot of reimbursements that nourishes the high-tech home care market?

Others worry about a different question of fairness. They are not concerned that we may be unfairly denying others access to more beneficial services foregone because home health care is provided. Rather, they worry that home services are appropriate only for a lucky fraction of the patients who might benefit medically from them.

Unless a family has personal and economic resources adequate to sustain a home clinic, a patient is not well served by being sent home. The concern is that some patients will be forced into homes incapable of receiving them, for cost-saving (and -shifting) reasons, and that other patients, who lack an adequate home setting, will be denied the benefits and be stuck in hospitals. For example, although a gay man with AIDS who is a well-educated professional may have resources, including friends or family, to provide the stable environment necessary to turn a home into a home clinic, the poor African American or Hispanic intravenous drug users, the fastest-growing group of patients with AIDS, will have no such personal resources and will be denied these benefits. The generous provision of a category of beneficial services to only some of the patients for whom they are medically suitable raises the question of whether fairness requires that all such patients get the services, including those for whom they are socially unsuitable.

I shall address these two questions of distributive justice. Answering the first question, that is, deciding whether it is fair to allocate new resources to these technologies, requires spelling out the conditions under which we should make rationing decisions of this sort. These conditions, I shall claim, are far from met in our health care system, and so any precipitous rationing decision of these services is likely to generate inequities rather than eliminate them. Rather than defend the status quo, however, I urge that we seek reforms that make it acceptable to undertake such rationing. Addressing the second question, the unfairness of giving these services to only the socially best-off patients who might benefit from them, also requires considering broader reforms of our social system.

I will set aside a further, difficult question, namely, how much we can or should use medical resources to redress broader social injustice.

Prerequisites for Rationing Fairly

To see whether justice requires or permits the rationing of high-tech home care, we must consider what justice in general says about the rationing of health care. For the sake of specificity, I shall draw on the fair equality of opportunity account I have developed in detail elsewhere (see Daniels 1985, 1988), although many of the points that follow do not presuppose that account. In this view, the central principle of justice that should govern the design of health care institutions, including institutions and procedures for limiting beneficial services, is a principle assuring fair equality of opportunity (see Rawls 1971; 1993, p. 184, n. 14).

The rationale for invoking this principle is that the central function of health care is to maintain and restore functioning that is normal or typical for our species. Disease and disability are construed as departures from species-typical functional organization (in short, normal functioning), and they shrink the range of opportunities open to an individual. More precisely, the normal opportunity range for a society is the array of plans of life that reasonable people in it can construct. An individual's fair share of the normal range is the array of life plans that individual can reasonably choose, given her or his talents and skills. This individual fair share is reduced when disease or disability affect an individual, but how serious the impairment is depends on the impact of the particular disease or disability. By aiming at preserving normal functioning, health care institutions thus make a significant but limited contribution to the protection of equality of opportunity.

It is important to accept the fact that resources are limited. Rawls (1971, pp. 126–27) called this moderate scarcity a "condition" of justice; if resources were abundant, we would not need principles to resolve conflicting claims on them. Although health care is specially important because of its impact on opportunity, it is not the only important good. Education, for example, competes with health care for resources that have a direct impact on fair equality of opportunity. So we must accept reasonable limits on health care resources. Specifically, resources do not permit everyone whose opportunities are diminished because of disease or disability to be restored to full functioning. We must pick and choose whose opportunities will be protected. Individual entitlements to health care are thus relative to the system: they are the result of resource-allocation choices made in a system aiming to abide by the equal opportunity principle (Daniels 1985, p. 54).

Justice requires, nevertheless, that we develop a public, fair procedure for deciding how health care institutions will allocate resources, given scarcity. This requirement amounts to rejecting the suggestion made by Calabresi and Bobbitt (1978) that the costs of making tragic choices explicitly are sometimes too high and that we might better appeal to implicit procedures. The point is that publicity is a crucial requirement of justice.

Ideally, the fair equality of opportunity principle would itself tell us specifically how to determine the moral priority among competing services and claims on them. Unfortunately, it offers only general and indeterminate advice (Daniels 1993, p. 225). It shares this feature with comparable distributive principles that govern other kinds of good (e.g., "equality before the law"). It tells us that disease and disabilities that more severely limit opportunities are more important to prevent or treat than less-disabling conditions and that therapies that effectively correct greater degrees of impairment are more important than ones that provide less benefit. But this advice is inadequate to decide crucial rationing questions.

At least four important types of problem are left unsolved (Daniels 1993 pp. 225–32), and all have some impact on our decisions about high-tech home care. First, there is the unsolved *priorities problem*. Although the equal-opportunity principle gives some priority to treating the most seriously ill or impaired individuals, since their opportunity is most compromised, it does not tell us just how much priority to give them. It would be implausible to act as maximizers, giving full priority to the worst-off cases, for that might require us to pour resources into those cases regardless of the size of the benefits (in opportunities) we forego for others. But in between giving no priority to the most seriously ill and giving full priority to them are myriad intermediary positions. We have no principled account of where to take our stand in the middle ground.

Second, there is the *aggregation problem*. We want resources to protect opportunity in the system as a whole, which implies that we should at least sometimes be able to aggregate more modest benefits to many people in ways that offset more significant benefits to few. But we are not straightforward maximizers of net benefit; we give some weight to producing more significant benefits for the most serious conditions. As with the priorities problem, however, no clear principled solution tells us where to take our stand in the middle ground.

Third, we are not sure how to weigh *fair chances* at obtaining some benefit against the importance of achieving *best outcomes*. No clear principle tells us just when we must compromise putting resources where they produce the greatest benefit and where we must respect each person's claim that she or he should have a chance at getting some benefit. Depending on the relative benefits in question, we may give more or less weight to fair chances or best outcomes. It is important to see that we have no principled solution to these problems at either an intuitive or a theoretical level (Daniels 1993, pp. 225–32).

Finally, we are not sure how much confidence to put in the outcome of a democratic decision procedure. The deepest form of this *democracy problem* derives from the fact that we cannot tell whether a democratic procedure should count as an instance of pure procedural justice or imperfect procedural justice. A fair spin of a roulette wheel determines a fair outcome: this is a case of pure procedural justice, since there is no prior notion of a fair outcome other than what the wheel determines. A criminal trial, however, is an imperfect procedure aimed at selecting all and only those who are guilty of committing the crime, and miscarriages of justice are infamous (see Rawls 1971, pp. 83–90). We are simply not sure whether the first three rationing problems have principled solutions. If they do, democratic procedures must aim at satisfying them; failure to satisfy them is grounds for criticizing the procedure, just as new evidence that someone is not guilty is grounds for criticizing the outcome of a trial. If there are no principled solutions to these problems, then whatever a fair democratic procedure yields will indeed determine what should count as fair.

I note in the next section how these unsolved problems bear on any decision regarding the use of high-tech home care, but here I want to continue elaborating the conditions under which fair rationing decisions may be made and implemented. Thus far I have argued that justice involves—requires—rationing and that we seek guidance from distributive principles, but we must at some level rely on a fair, democratic procedure that makes the grounds for choice publicly accessible. I want to emphasize two other conditions.

To make judgments about the relative importance—medical and moral—of high-tech home care services, we must have reasonably *adequate information* about its costs and benefits, as well as about the costs and benefits of other kinds of services competing with them for resources. The decision to use one kind of service rather than another is a decision about *opportunity costs*. Here I intend the double entendre. In the standard economic sense, in using resources for one kind of therapy we must compare the net benefits of alternative therapies, considering the benefits we forego when we use one service rather than another and not just whether one therapy has a net benefit considered by itself. The double meaning is that we are considering alternative impacts on the normal opportunity range: the foregone benefits are a cost to the opportunities of others.

The remaining condition has a bearing on the design of the institutions in which rationing decisions will be carried out. Rationing choices should be made within what I (loosely) call a *closed system* (Daniels 1986, pp. 1381–82). A system is closed if the resources relevant to decisions made within it are determinate and the costs and benefits of the decisions about resource allocation made in it are internal to it. For example, if we decide to forego one service in favor of another, then the cost of foregoing it is born by those in the system, and the benefits and costs of the alternative are as well.

A closed system forces us to face the consequences of our deliberate choices to deny benefits to some people who have reasonable claims on them. To see why this is important, consider two examples in which the system is not closed. Suppose we are a managed care system and that we agree that we should not make certain high-tech home care services available because, compared with alternative uses of the resources, we should provide other services instead. Suppose further, however, that instead of putting the resources we save into the preferred alternative, we simply put them toward bonuses for the medical staff. The costs and benefits of what we actually do are not factored into our original decision: the closed system has leaked. Similarly, suppose we decide that Medicaid should not provide certain high-tech home services because adding them will increase the rate of growth of Medicaid budgets and because alternative uses of the resources have greater benefits. Nevertheless, these services not covered by Medicaid are then covered by private insurance or can be bought out of pocket by those wealthy enough. The system again has a leak: our denial of the service on the grounds that the opportunity cost of offering it is too great has been superseded by a different rationing principle, availability by ability to pay. A judgment that might be sufficient to justify a rationing choice in a closed system (namely, a comparison of opportunity costs) may not be sufficient if a different rationing principle operates by default in the "leaky" system as a whole.

Rationing High-Tech Home Care

On the face of it, none of these conditions that are prerequisite for rationing fairly is met in the current situation, and any decision to target categorically high-tech home care for rationing seems unjustifiable. Specifically, we have no public, fair democratic procedure for deciding whether or how to ration these high-tech services. In addition, any rationing choices we now make fail to apply in a closed system: we have a mixed public-private system of payments with no global budget constraining resources. Finally, we lack adequate information about the costs and benefits of these technologies, and we lack comparable information about the technologies competing for the same resources. Each of these claims warrants further explanation, and I will take them in reverse order.

As I noted earlier, one force driving the growth of high-tech home care services is the belief that it is less expensive to deliver infusion therapy, for example, at home than in the hospital. Three key assumptions underlie this judgment: similar medical benefits and risks obtain in both situations; delivering these technologies in the hospital involves charges that include the reasonable overhead involved in maintaining a hospital facility; and the overhead costs of running a household clinic will not be chargeable to third-party payers. Each assumption warrants comment.

First, though I cannot give evidence for the claim, I think we know less than is assumed about the actual comparability of medical benefits and risks in the two settings. We probably have not run controlled trials comparing outcomes in a way that could lead to a precise calculation of comparable risks. Nevertheless, let the first assumption stand.

Second, hospital charges often reflect far more than the real costs of a service. For example, hospitals factor into their charges an allowance for future hospital expansion, for debt-servicing of past, unrelated capital investments, for investment in new technologies, and, in the case of for-profit institutions, even for profits that will be spent on nonmedical investments. Practically speaking, however inflated, these are the charges a third-party payer must take into account, but the charges clearly distort our view about the real costs of a service. They stack the deck in favor of funneling new resources into home care services.

Third, the costs of home delivery of these services are distorted in opposite directions. On the one hand, they are clearly underestimated. Although it may be reasonable from the perspective of a private third-party insurer to omit the true costs to a household of sustaining a patient at home, since these will not show up as charges, these social costs are real and ought to play a role in rationing decisions. The societal and family costs may be quite significant: lost earning power, the cost of replacing trained workers, costs to children from having parents deeply enmeshed in providing home care, the loss of family mobility. Ignoring these costs yields judgments that reflect the interests of the third-party payer while not adequately capturing the societal perspective.

Since rationing decisions are matters of justice, I believe they should reflect societal concerns about how to meet obligations and should not simply constitute a form of cost-shifting—unless the principle behind the cost-shifting is itself publicly defended as a rationing principle. Another way to think about the point is to suggest that we have failed to close the system within which the calculation about costs and benefits is made; crucial costs fall outside the subsystem within which third-party payers are making their decisions, yet the broader view captures facts necessary for a societal decision about rationing. Some problems of this sort are unavoidable in a decentralized system, but some are features we get because we fail to link the components of our system into a true system.

Other forces work to overstate the real costs of high-tech home care, namely, the failures to force the reasonable pricing of these services either through regulation or through appropriate negotiation with a properly designed purchasing agent. Paralleling the distorting effects we noticed in the case of hospital charges, we have the dramatic pricing effects documented by New York City Consumer Affairs Commissioner Mark Green (City of New York DCA 1991). Home care providers selling services to third-party payers in New York often refuse to detail their charges and the justification for them in advance. There are no standards for how such charges are made. For example, infusion companies typically charge for nursing when many AIDS patients prefer self-administration. There are wide variations in charges from company to company, so much so that there is no real relationship between charges and actual costs, and markups can approach 600 percent. The effect is enormous. Green (City of New York DCA 1991, p. 13) claimed that costs for total parenteral nutrition (TPN) account for nearly one-third of the estimated $150,000 average lifetime cost of caring for an AIDS patient. In the face of gross profiteering, made possible because the purchasing system fails to act as a unified buyer of services with the power to negotiate for uniform practices and reasonable charges, we really cannot say much about the relative savings that accrue from substituting high-tech home care for hospital-based services.

One last point bears on our knowledge about costs. There are no large-scale studies of the degree to which home services act as substitutes for hospital services and the degree to which they constitute an additional utilization. For example, individuals who might reconcile themselves to dying at home without intensive therapies might accept home treatments they would refuse in a hospital setting. Without knowing whether this phenomenon is small or large, we cannot say how much home services save money.

A proper rationing decision must rest on reasonably good information about the relative costs and benefits of the services being compared. So far, I have said we lack that information even about comparisons of home and hospital delivery of the same technologies. But we should not really be comparing home and hospital delivery of the same technologies as a basis for rationing categories of care. Rather, rationing requires an appropriate comparison of all technologies competing for the limited resources. Targeting high-tech home care for rationing just because it is new is arbitrary from the perspective of fair rationing policy. Rather, we must compare both high-tech home care *and* hospital delivery of the same services with a broader set of services.

As soon as we see this point, it is obvious that we must distinguish the quite different types of benefit delivered by various high-tech home services. Some technologies (for example, home infusion of antibiotics) may cure an acute episode of infection. For some patients, this may produce long life of high quality. For others, it may buy only a few months or weeks of life of diminished quality before death. Similar points may be made about TPN, which sometimes produces only palliation during a prolonged dying process, but which can be part of a more beneficial curing process. Simply lumping together all services as "high tech" or as "home delivered" completely ignores the *relevant* differences for the purposes of rationing decisions.

Once we sort out the relevant contrasts among the uses of these technologies, whether delivered at home or in a hospital, we still have a task that involves unsolved moral issues of the sort I noted earlier. There will be patients who are very seriously ill, with terrible prognoses, for whom some high-tech home service (or hospital service) would yield only very modest benefit at significant cost. Should we simply seek to produce comparable or greater benefits at lower cost for patients who are initially less seriously ill, or should we be so concerned about helping those whose prospects are worst that we forego producing more cost-effective benefits elsewhere? Should we, for example, devote respirator technologies to patients in a persistent vegetative state (PVS), accepting that the prolongation of their comatose state is a medical benefit? Or should we be willing to aggregate benefits that fall well short of extending life to other patients and conclude that these aggregated benefits are more important to deliver than the benefit to the PVS patient? We lack principled solutions to these and to the other problems I noted earlier, yet nearly every comparison of a use of high-tech home care with uses of other services for other categories of patients will involve one or another unsolved rationing problem. I will return to this issue shortly when I talk about the importance of relying on a fair democratic process for making rationing decisions.

The fact that we do not operate our health care system as a closed system for the purposes of rationing has major implications for this discussion of rationing high-tech home care. I am going to operationalize—and simplify—the idea of a closed system by considering a globally budgeted health care system and contrasting it with ours. Under a global budget, expenditures made for one type of service will not be available for others. In contrast, in our open system, "leaks" permit new resources to be added, when we think of the system as a whole, despite the decision made by one party or sector to restrict the use of a service. A leaky system means we do not really live with the consequences of our rationing decisions. Though I have touched on some of these points, let me emphasize three implications.

A global budget forces decisionmakers to face the consequences of their choices. One important use of high-tech home care services will be for seriously disabled infants who need respirator, infusion, or monitoring services. The costs of these services should be considered as the downstream costs of aggressive treatment of low-birthweight or otherwise seriously defective neonates. A decision to reduce the availability of these services should be factored into the related decisions whether to use aggressive rescue efforts for the neonates. A system in which the costs of these services are borne within different budgets (for example, by different insurers) means that we are not really forced to face the consequences of decisions made separately within the different budgets. For example, if public budgets largely cover the costs of seriously disabled children, but aggressive rescue efforts are decided on by those who must contend primarily with private insurers or even with different public budgets, then those who authorize aggressive rescue efforts can escape its consequences.

A closed system means that rationing decisions are not converted into cost-shifting exercises and that services foregone to direct resources into a more important service actually have that effect. I have already noted that the decision to favor high-tech home delivery over hospital delivery of these services involves shifting costs to families. Suppose, however, that public insurance no longer included coverage for a broad range of high-tech home care services. It might even be the case that the basis for this decision was reasonable in the light of the comparison of benefits and costs of certain uses of these services compared with other uses of resources. Some of these services might still be covered by private insurers, and some would still be purchased out-of-pocket by some families. We will not have redirected resources in the way intended by the decision, at least not when we look at the system as a whole.

Finally, the lack of a global budget can often mean that someone responsible for a rationing decision might make it on grounds that seem reasonable, given the opportunity costs of relevant competitors for the use of the resources, but in the system as a whole the operative rationing principle might be the ability to pay. For example, if some services were excluded from a "basic" benefit package in a national health insurance system that contained competing private insurers, but these services were available in more deluxe plans that cost more, then only those willing and able to afford the more deluxe package will be able to obtain the benefits. If only the best-off individuals can get these services, we might complain that there was an objectionable inequality, but it might not be thought so serious. But if the worst-off groups are denied these services, while they are obtainable by most other individuals, then the *structure of inequality* that results from the rationing decision is objectionable (Daniels 1986; 1991, pp. 2233–34). In effect, some effects of relying on the ability to pay are worse than others.

The remaining condition for fair rationing, the requirement that there be a fair democratic process for making rationing decisions, is not met in most health care systems. Even comprehensive, globally budgeted systems like the Canadian system lack an attempt to articulate publicly the grounds for key decisions bearing on the allocation of health care resources. Many European systems are struggling to articulate and justify principles that they can use to guide rationing choices (Government Committee 1992). I would like to illustrate the virtue of a public, democratic process by referring to Oregon's ongoing attempt to establish priorities among health care services.

When Oregon developed a list of 709 ranked condition/treatment pairs in 1991, it drew considerable criticism for the very low ranking given to the treatment of HIV-infection for AIDS patients with less than six months to live. That ranking might be thought (incorrectly) to bear on the rationing of high-tech home services, like infusion therapies so widely used by AIDS patients. Was Oregon simply denying those therapies to these patients?

According to the executive director of the Oregon Health Services Commission, Paige Sipes-Metzler (personal communication, January 1993), many of the uses of these technologies would in fact be permitted. For example, the infusion of antibiotics was really categorized as the treatment of a specific opportunistic infection, and that use of high-tech home care would have been covered by a condition-treatment pair ranked much higher on the list. Similarly, TPN for a terminally ill AIDS patient would have been covered as "palliative" care and thus not rationed out of the system by the low ranking of item 709 either. In fact, all that the Health Service Commission intended was that aggressive treatment of the HIV infection itself for late-stage HIV patients not be authorized, given that no effective treatment was available.

The treatment condition pair ranked 709 has been eliminated from the version of Oregon's plan submitted in November 1992 for Medicaid waiver. According to Sipes-Metzler, experts testified that there was little basis for singling out late-stage HIV infection as a well-defined stage of a disease. The point of having made a public, explicit decision of the sort made in 1991, in the context of an accountable, democratic process, is that further criticism was able to lead to a change. Since the grounds for the decision were public, they could be publicly challenged.

A public, democratic process that undertook to consider whether to ration certain high-tech home care services would have to defend its decisions along many of the dimensions I have articulated. It would have to show that its cost and benefit estimates were reasonable; that process might bring public scrutiny to bear on the kinds of abuses Green (City of New York DCA 1991) documented in the home care services industry. It would have to make appropriate comparisons of competitor services: only a much more fine-grained assessment than one that uses such clumsy categories as "high tech" and "home versus hospital" would survive scrutiny. Finally, the process would require taking a stand on the moral choices I earlier categorized as "unsolved rationing problems." Some particular stance would have to be adopted on how much priority should be given the sickest patients, as well as on how we should aggregate benefits. Either we would be forced to develop a principled defense of the stance we adopt on these issues or we would simply fall back on the claim that since there was no consensus on principle, it was sufficient to have democratic agreement. Either result would be ethically defensible.

I do not mean to imply that we should adopt the Oregon strategy of trying to rank broadly construed treatment/condition pairs. There are many reasons to think that we might ultimately have to rely on gatekeeping decisions by clinicians who make much more finely tuned assessments in the light of information they have about their particular patients' conditions and prognoses. For example, Canadian practitioners appear to exclude some categories of patients, or patients sufficiently unlikely to derive benefit, from ICUs more than do their U.S. counterparts (Daniels and Sabin, unpublished research). They may have internalized a somewhat more restrictive approach to the use of ICUs because they operate in a more restrictive, globally constrained environment. I do not believe their practice is guided by adequate public discussion of the kinds of decision they make: here they lack a fair democratic process, as do all systems. But the approach, relying on the internalized judgment of practitioners who have to negotiate how their patients are placed in a globally constrained setting, is an alternative to the Oregon arrangement, an alternative that would be vastly improved with the assistance of a public democratic process.

Social Barriers to the Use of High-Tech Home Care

Suppose for the sake of argument that we have met the conditions necessary for making a fair rationing decision and that we have decided that certain high-tech home care services ought to be reimbursable in our insurance scheme. We might in fact suppose that there is a strong justification for making the corresponding hospital versions of these services less available or even unavailable for those who are medically suitable. For example, though the home versions are cost-effective beyond some threshold we can agree on, the hospital delivery fails to meet the threshold. Were there only hospital versions of these technologies, they would not be included in the system. The questions of fairness we now face concern those who are medically suitable for these services but whose home situation makes their provision inappropriate.

One way to face hard choices is to duck them by finding an alternative. If hospital-based versions of a therapy fail to meet some criterion for inclusion, whereas home versions should be included, then there may also be an intermediary format for delivering the service that might also warrant inclusion. Some group setting or low-overhead nursing home setting might meet the relevant criteria. Then the issue would be whether the health care system is designed so that such settings will be made available. Another alternative might be to provide additional nursing care in whatever home setting would otherwise be unsuitable. But this alternative may push the costs over the relevant threshold, or it may be unavailable because of the serious inadequacies of the home setting.

Clearly there will be some cases we cannot duck in this way. The general form of the problem is this: reasonable rationing criteria mean that some medically suitable people (specifically, those who are worst off economically or socially) will be left unprotected by the system in cases when economically or socially more fortunate individuals can be helped. In effect, we are allowing better-off individuals to use their extra resources to subsidize the delivery of a service they would otherwise also be denied, since it is unavailable in the hospital for them as well. When different benefits are available to people through more expensive insurance plans or out of pocket, we have a multitiered system. What are the moral implications of such tiers?

How we should respond to this situation depends, I think, on the kind of benefit the service in question provides. If it has a significant effect on individuals, that is, it protects the opportunity range in a significant way, then I think the tiering that results in the system is seriously objectionable. This is precisely what is prohibited in the Dutch and German systems, where private and public insurance schemes rarely differ in anything but amenities or other nonmedically necessary services. If, however, the benefits of the high-tech home services were really this great, then it is less likely that the original rationing criteria would have had the consequences we are supposing. It is more likely that the benefits are modest or marginal; in that case, we can tolerate better the structure of inequality that results from the hypothetical rationing.

A compromise outcome might be this: if the benefit is significant (which of course we would need to define), but it would be far more cost effective to deliver that benefit at home, then we might provide hospital delivery for those for whom we can find no more cost-effective alternative (even though hospital delivery considered by itself would not have been included in reasonable rationing criteria). Under a global budget, this decision would have opportunity costs, and we would have to make sure we were not protecting equality of opportunity in this instance at the cost of a more serious sacrifice of it elsewhere. Alas, being precise at this point is difficult, because many of the judgments depend on what the alternative uses of resources might turn out to be. What counts as a "significant benefit," for instance, is a judgment we can make only when we are considering what options really are feasible alternatives under the circumstances.

In short, to the question of how we should react to the inequity that arises between patients for whom high-tech home care is suitable and those for whom it is not, we must respond: it depends. It depends on how significant the benefits are, what alternatives are available, and on whether reducing this inequity creates more significant ones elsewhere. More specific answers are possible only when we have very specific cases and alternatives in mind.

Conclusions

We have seen how the rapid growth of high-tech home care—
brought sharply into public discussion because of the applicability of
many of these high-tech services to those suffering from AIDS—
raises two general questions about the just distribution of health-care
resources. First, some people believe that we provide far too many
high-cost services that produce only marginal benefits and that where
we see a costly new category of such services emerging we should act
boldly to restrict its dissemination. Doing so is what fairness to other
patients elsewhere in the system requires.

In response to this first issue, I have argued that we must meet
certain conditions before we can make *any* rationing judgments fairly.
Our decisions about rationing must be made as a result of a fair, democratic process. The process must make public the principles and reasons underlying rationing decisions, and decisions must rest on an
adequate basis of information about outcomes and costs for the relevant comparison class of alternative services. The decisions must
apply within systems that are appropriately closed; otherwise, a rationing decision made on one set of grounds (comparisons of benefits
and costs) is converted into another (availability by the ability to pay).
The ability to pay may sometimes be acceptable, but only in a highly
restricted set of circumstances.

I conclude that these conditions are not met now, and that any
precipitous decision to ration a whole category of services—high tech
or home care—is indefensible. We must, however, reform our system
so that specific rationing decisions of the relevant sort *can* be made.
We can ration fairly only in the context of a system that in general
conforms to requirements of justice, and our system is very far from
that.

The second issue of fairness concerns the inequity that results
when only the best-off sectors of society have access to the benefits
of high-tech home care. I have argued that how serious this inequity
is depends on the difference in benefits that results. Where significant
benefits are denied to worst-off groups, we risk failing to protect
equality of opportunity; we should then seek alternatives that keep
inequalities within acceptable limits.

REFERENCES

Calabresi, G., and Bobbitt, P. 1978. *Tragic Choices.* New York: Norton.
Callahan, D. 1987. *Setting Limits: Medical Goals in an Aging Society.* New
York: Simon & Schuster.

Daniels, N. 1985. *Just Health Care*. Cambridge: Cambridge University Press.

——. 1986. Why saying no to patients in the United States is so hard: Cost containment, justice, and provider autonomy. *New England Journal of Medicine* 314:1281–83.

——. 1988. *Am I My Parents' Keeper?: An Essay on Justice between the Young and the Old*. New York: Oxford University Press.

——. 1991. Is the Oregon rationing plan fair? *JAMA* 265: 2232–35.

——. 1993. Rationing fairly: Programmatic considerations. *Bioethics* 7:224–33.

Daniels, N., and Sabin, J. Unpublished research (case studies and interviews) with hospital personnel in Toronto. Research sponsored by Robert Wood Johnson Foundation, in progress.

Government Committee on Choices in Health Care. 1992. *Choices in Health Care*. Netherlands: Ministry of Welfare, Health and Cultural Affairs.

City of New York, Department of Consumer Affairs (DCA). 1991. *Making a Killing on AIDS: Home Health Care and Pentamidine*, May.

Mehlman, M., and Youngner, S.J. 1991. *Delivering High Technology Home Care*. New York: Springer.

Rawls, J. 1971. *A Theory of Justice*. Cambridge, Mass.: Harvard University Press.

——. 1993. *Political Liberalism*. New York: Columbia University Press.

Index

Italic *f* following page number denotes figure; italic *t* following page number denotes table.

Ability to pay principle, 237, 241, 246, 248–49, 250
Abuse: adult, 187–89; domestic, 169–72; elder, 137, 185–86; in hospitals, 169–72; potential for, in assisted suicide, 177
Access, 28; justice and, 235–51
Accommodation of interests, 21
Accountability, 209, 211, 217, 230
Acquired immune-deficiency syndrome (AIDS)/AIDS patients, 8, 15, 27, 38, 79–90, 105, 160–61, 224, 228, 250; case management services for, 231; costs of care with, 222–24; and home care market, 24, 235; managing costs of, 230; rationing care for, 246–47; treatment of, 227, 237
Adult abuse and neglect, 187–89
Advance directives, 116, 123, 182–84, 187–88, 189
Age: of care recipient and caregiver, 136–37; and dependency, 109
Aggregation problem, 239, 244, 247
Aging services, 204
AIDS-related complex (ARC), 80, 81
Alternatives to home care, 18, 22–23, 26, 28, 46–47, 87, 248
American Medical Association (AMA), 13; home care guidelines, 181, 213
Antibiotic therapies, 87, 221, 231, 244; for AIDS patients, 246; costs of, 226; intravenous, 110, 116–17
Antibiotics, 67, 92, 93, 107; administration of, 71–73
Antiretroviral therapy, 81
Appropriateness: of discharge, 136, 138–39; of services, 43, 93, 236–37, 248–49
Appropriateness criteria, 211
Assisted suicide, 92–93, 176–77
Autonomy (patient), 21, 22, 102, 108,

123, 166, 183; threats to, 172; in treatment decisions, 187
Autopsy, 191, 192
AZT (zidovudine), 81, 82

Beds, air-fluidized, 107, 109, 111–13
Benefits/burdens, 4–5, 16, 20, 27, 29, 144; and cancer patients, 74–76; information about, 17–18; of respirators and TPN, 41–43; with technology-dependent children, 47–48
Benefits/liabilities: home vs. hospital care, 242; and rationing, 249, 250; in terminal illness, 99–105, 100*t*. *See also* Costs/benefits
Best interests standard, 14, 18, 21; in treatment decisions, 189, 190
Blue Cross/Blue Shield, 88, 230
Bolus feedings, 71, 100, 114–15
Bone marrow transplant, 72
Bowel dysfunction/obstruction, 71, 84, 115

Cachexia, 84, 115
Cancer, 8, 38, 65–78, 105; and elderly patients, 130–35; immune-deficiency-related, 80; therapies with, 65, 66
Capacity to care: suffering and, 153–62
Capitated programs, 205
Cardiopulmonary resuscitation (CPR), 188–89
Care, 107, 149; continuum of, 199, 231; coordination of, 10; duration of, 2, 11
Care companions, 174, 175
Care plan, 29, 181–82
Caregiver(s), 2, 29, 92; age of, 136–37; AIDS patients, 85, 87; burdens to, 6–9, 11, 12, 22, 74, 75; capacities and projects of, 155–58; concern for personhood of, 18, 19; elderly, 19–20, 136–37; evaluation of, 153–62;

Caregiver(s) *(continued)*
  fatigue in, 96–98; isolation of, 104; paid, 10; and pain management, 95–96; relationship with patient, 153–55; support for, 138; at risk for psychological problems, 99
Caregiving: case studies of, 153; compensated, 199; length of, 136, 137–38; women and, 155, 156–57
Caremark, 231
Caring, 7–8, 26; justice within, 18–22
Case management, 11, 13, 28, 29, 204
Case management services, 231
Catheterization, urinary tract, 109, 113–14
Catheters, 1, 39, 67–69, 73, 81, 107; problems with, 40–41, 120; transtracheal oxygen administration, 121–22
Chemotherapy, 69, 70, 71–73, 83, 87
Children, 7, 75, 170; "best interests" of, 14; costs of care for, 43–45; disabled, 245; and moral worth, 61; parents caring for, 157; and problems of identity, 5, 6; as "silent sufferers," 99; TPN for, 35, 38–41; values and, 59; ventilator-dependent, 8, 9, 11, 19, 35–38, 41, 42, 44, 45, 53–54. *See also* Technology-dependent children
Chimeras, 53–56, 61–62
Chronic illness, 227–28, 230, 231
Chronic obstructive pulmonary disease (COPD), 122, 123
Closed system(s), 240–41, 244–45, 250
Cognitive function/capacity, 99; in elderly, 129, 136; and nutritional support, 115–16; and right to make treatment decisions, 186
Communication, 17–18, 105, 141–43, 144; deficiencies of, 9, 11
Community-based care, 28, 227
Computerized ambulatory infusion device, 117
Congressional committees, 28–29
Consent, informed and freely given, 17–18, 22–23, 213; emergency exception to, 190
Consumer satisfaction, 210–11, 212
Continuous ambulatory peritoneal dialysis (CAPD), 110, 119–21
Contracts, 22, 23
Coroner, 191
Cost containment, 15, 108, 123, 156, 160–61, 224, 225–28, 235–36; and early discharge, 138

Cost-effectiveness, 24–25, 27, 161, 198–99, 226–28, 231, 244, 248, 249; hospital homelike care, 175
Cost reduction, 150
Cost shifting, 236, 242–43, 245
Costs, 1, 12, 28, 29, 102–3, 160; in care of elderly, 111, 112, 113, 114, 115, 117, 118, 120, 122, 124; in care of technology-dependent children, 43, 44–45, 48, 60; direct, 221–22; to family, 187; home care, relative to hospital, 24–25, 43, 44–45, 74, 75, 92, 198–99, 214–15, 226–28, 242–43, 248; of medical care, 149; of TPN, 71
Costs/benefits, 26, 27, 250; need for information about, 240, 241; and rationing, 247
Cultural factors, 140–41, 176
Cytomegalovirus infection, 72, 80, 221

Death, 99, 104; home/hospital, 175–78
Decision for home care, 93–95; medical and ethical indications, 16–23; open to renegotiation, 23, 47
Decision making, 144; home as site of, 180–87; patients and families in, 108, 142; regulations regarding, 182–83; surrogate, 189–90
Decubitus care, 109, 111–13
Dehydration, 70, 116
Delivery systems, 197, 198, 217; failures of, 9–12; fragmentation of, 205–7
Demand/supply forces, 235, 236
Dementia, 80, 82, 115–16
Democratic process, 239–40, 241, 244, 246–48, 250
Dependency, 44, 100–101, 109, 170
Depression, 140
Development (child), 56, 58
Diagnosis-related groups (DRGs), 11, 108, 112, 226–27
Dialysis, 107, 197, 110, 119–21
Discharge: appropriateness of, 136, 138–39; early 14–15, 20
Discharge-planning, 9, 14, 17, 123, 139; HIV/AIDS patients, 86–87
Discharging patients "sicker and quicker," 15, 91, 108, 117, 138, 166
Disease progression, 8, 85, 95–96
Distributive justice, 237–49, 250
Do Not Resuscitate (DNR) orders, 188, 189, 193
Domestic abuse, 169–72
Double agency, 14–15
Drug administration, 71–73
Drug infusion, 67

Durable medical equipment, 207, 208, 228
Duty, 18–22, 151, 152, 162
Dying at home, 3, 66, 175–76; cases, 180–85, 187–91; problems and protocols for, 180–96; public policy recommendations, 192–93
Dying patient(s), 8, 94–95. *See also* Terminal illness

Economic impact, 220–34
Elder abuse and neglect, 137, 184–85
Elderly (the), 92–93, 125, 198, 214, 235; cancer in, 65–66; and dying at home, 177–78; high-tech care for, 107–28; high-tech care for, case studies, 129–35, 137, 138, 139, 140, 141–43, 144; impact of care on, 136–39; issues in care for, 136–39; in Medicare HMOs, 205; recommendations for care of, 139–44; sickroom for, 159
Elderly parents, responsibility for care of, 149, 150–51, 154–55
Emergencies, 100, 110
Emergency alarms, 1, 109, 110–11
Emergency services/squads, 46, 102, 189, 192, 193
Empire Blue Cross/Blue Shield, 223, 224, 226, 230
End-stage renal disease (ESRD) program, 201
Enteral feeding, 70, 71, 109, 114–16, 221
Equality of opportunity, 27, 237–41, 249, 250
Ethic of care, 18, 19, 151–52, 163–64
Ethical issues, 1–31; in care of elderly, 112–13, 118, 123–24; in death at home, 192, 193; in home care of terminally ill, 91–106; post-death, 191–92; with technology-dependent children, 55–56
Ethics committees, 192
Euthanasia, 92–93, 160, 176

Fair chances/best outcomes, 239
Fairness, questions of, 235–37, 248–49
Familial duties, limits of, 18–22
Family(ies), 3, 12, 28, 29, 92, 94, 105; benefits burdens of home care, 7, 74, 75; costs to, 227, 236, 242; and death at home, 175–76; of elderly persons, 136–39; evaluation of, 94–95; home care agency and, 187–89; in hospital-based medicine, 12–13; impact of high-tech care on, 4–12;

nurse functions assumed by, 216; and problems of identity, 5–6; and quality assurance, 209; relationship with care providers and patients, 12–16; support for, 193; of technology-dependent children, 43, 44, 45, 47; and treatment decisions, 142, 186–87, 189–91
Family compensation/reimbursement, 199, 206, 217
Family relationships, 140–41, 167, 171; impact of illness on, 172, 173
Fatigue (caregiver), 96–98
Feeding devices/tubes, 92, 93, 197. *See also* Nasogastric feeding tube
Feminist perspective, 149, 155, 172
Financial considerations: in control over dying, 177. *See also* Funding
Financial resources, 67, 94, 102–3, 117; third-party payment, 224–25
Flexible benefits plan(s), 155, 159
For-profit companies, 20, 23–24, 206, 230
Foster care system, 46
Friendship-based duties, limits of, 18–22
Functional impairment, 109, 203. *See also* Cognitive function/capacity
Functional status, 136–37
Funding, 45; fragmentation of, 200–205

Gastrointestinal tract, 70, 71, 84, 107, 221; infections of, 80
Gastrostomy, 71, 84, 100–101
Gatekeeping decisions, 107, 247–48
Geriatric home care: historical perspective, 107–9; technologies in, 109–25
Global budget(s), 245–46, 249
Guilt, 20, 102, 104, 157

Harm, risk of, 197–98
Health care policy, 105, 150, 183; money-driven, 28; response to need in, 163–64
Health care professionals, 140; and home care, 14–16, 74–75; paternalism by, 170–71; role of, 77, 95
Health care providers: liability risks, 212–13; licensing (proposed), 230; procedural obligations, 182–83; and quality assurance, 209, 211–12; relationship with patients and caregivers, 12–16; standards for, 228
Health care reform: ageism in, 124–25
Health care system, 27–28
Health expenditures, 26, 222f, 228, 229f

Health maintenance organizations (HMOs), 205, 206, 207
Helen House, 158
Hemodialysis, 119, 120
High-tech home care: appeal of, 224–25; components in, 207–8; in context, 197–219; dangers of, 197–98; defined, 197–98, 221–22; and dying at home, 180–96; economic impact of, 220–34; ethical and social implications of, 1–31; for HIV/AIDS patients, 87–88; issues and trends in, 213–17; quality issues specific to, 212–13; rationing, 241–48; skeptical challenge to, 26–27; social and psychological burdens of, 42–43; social barriers to use of, 248–49
"High touch" care, 25, 75, 236
HIV. See Human immunodeficiency virus (HIV) patients
HIV-related complications, 81–84
Home, 4, 22, 166; death at, 175–78; as decision-making site, 180–87; paternalism and abuses in, 169–72; patients' preference for, 74, 91; stereotypes of, 167–68; terminal care at, 91–93; transformation of, 166–79
Home care, 108, 221; barriers to, 16–17; elsewhere than at home, 174–75; expenditures for, 222f; forces driving growth of, 235–36; vs. nursing homes, 215–16; organization of, 199–208; outcomes for, 76, 210–11; policies and procedures for organization of, 183–84; prerequisites to, 45–46; quality assurance, 209; trial basis, 21–22
Home care advisors, 157–58, 161
Home care agencies/health agencies, 13, 92, 109, 129; and accountability, 209; certified, 88; and death at home, 181–85; delivery of services, 205, 206; ethics committees, 192; and family(ies), 187–89; and insurance, 204–5; and Medicaid, 203; Medicare-certified, 201–2, 205, 206; patient screening by, 229–30; post-death issues, 191–92; problems with, 133–35, 138, 143; quality of care, 144; services provided by, 105, 204–5; specialized, 205, 214; and treatment decisions, 190; written policies and procedures, 182, 192
Home care industry/companies, 108; abuses in, 247; fear of malpractice lawsuits, 185; growth of, 222–28,

231–32, 242, 250; home intravenous care, 117; Medicare and, 201; pricing practices, 228–31; profit motive/profits, 20, 74, 76; services provided by, 25, 66–67; specialized, 198, 205, 206, 207, 208
Home care plan(s), 45, 94, 95
Home care workers, 156. See also Health care professionals
Home environment: erosion of, 103–4; facilities in, 158–60; inadequate, inappropriate, 227, 237, 248–49
Home parenteral nutrition (HPN), 84, 115–16
Home visits, 15–16, 143, 200
Homeless people, 86–87, 167, 174, 178
Hospice(s)/hospice care, 10, 102, 172, 177, 201, 210
Hospice movement, 91, 175
Hospital-to-home transfers, 7, 166, 172
Hospitalizations: with AIDS, 80; for cancer patients, 70, 72
Hospitals, 12–13, 199, 200, 220, 236; death at, 175–78; exposure to infectious disease in, 66; hidden costs to, in shift to home care, 227; home care at, 174–75; paternalism and abuses in, 169–72; stereotypes of, 167–68; transforming, 166–79; when preferable to home, 173–74
Housekeeping assistance, 7, 159, 202, 204, 221
Housing needs, 159, 163
Human-and-machine combinations, 53, 55–56, 61
Human immunodeficiency virus (HIV) patients, 79–90, 235; rationing care for, 247; treatment of, 220, 221, 223
Hydration, 67, 70–71, 84, 116

Identity, problems of, 5–6
Immune deficiency, 79, 80
Infection(s), 67, 117; in AIDS patients, 80, 82; in cancer patients, 72; catheters and, 40–41, 69; in elderly, 116, 123. See also Opportunistic infections
Information, 142, 213; about benefits/burdens, 17–18; need for, 28–29, 240, 241, 250
Infusion companies, specialized, 205, 206, 207, 208
Infusion feedings, 71, 100–101
Infusion pumps, 1, 13–14, 67, 72, 92; for analgesics, 93, 107, 118; for feeding, 114–15; for PCA, 110, 118

Infusion therapy(ies), 197, 221–22, 225; for AIDS patients, 246–47; for cancer patients, 72; cost of, 222, 226, 246; not covered by Medicare, 207–8; payment rates for (proposed), 230
Infusion therapy market, 222, 223*f*, 235; costs and markups, 229*t*
In-Home Supportive Services (IHSS), 204
Insurance, 15, 67, 102, 117, 204–5, 231, 249; and cancer patients, 76; and care of technology-dependent children, 43; and HIV/AIDS patients, 86, 88; and home health agencies, 230; services covered by, 75, 111, 224–25, 245, 246
Insurance companies, 9–10, 23, 37, 215
Interdisciplinary team(s), 181–82
Intermediate care facilities, 11, 46–47
Intravenous therapy, 67–69, 73, 81, 87, 110, 116–17

Jejunostomy, 71, 84, 100–101
Justice, 18–22, 235–51

Kantian ethics, 151–52, 162, 164
Kaposi sarcoma (KS), 79, 80, 82–83
Kidney failure, 110, 119–21

Legal issues: in death at home, 176–77, 192, 193; post-death, 192–93; in responsibility for care, 150–51
Liability risks, 190, 212–13
Life expectancy, 108–9, 125, 161
Life-sustaining treatment: family and, 190–91, 193; right to refuse, 171–72, 185–86
Long-term care, 22, 25, 203

Malignancies, 82–83
Malpractice lawsuits, 185
Market/marketing (health care), 23, 24, 25, 28, 29, 47, 116; infusion therapy, 222, 223*f*, 235
Medic Alert, 111
Medicaid, 88, 102–3, 111, 182, 184, 202–3, 207, 214, 230, 241; coverage, 225; funding for ventilator-dependent children, 37–38
Medicaid waivers, 38, 45, 203–4, 213, 225, 247
Medical care, dehumanization of, 108
Medical equipment and supplies, cost of, 222

Medical examiners, 102, 191
Medical management: of HIV infection/ AIDS, 81–84
Medicalization of the home, 2–4
Medicare, 61, 75, 88, 102, 111, 112, 135, 182; cost-containment, 123; HMOs, 205; home health care, 200–202; prepayment system, 108; services covered/not covered, 117, 207–8, 225
Medicare: beneficiaries, 213–14; carriers, 228
Medications, cost of, 221–22
Memorial Sloan-Kettering Psychiatry Service Home Care Program, 94
Mental health care providers, 86
Metaphor, 53, 55, 61
Money, 15; and moral worth, 60–61
Monitoring, 76, 117, 123, 197, 235
Moral obligation: collective, 160, 162–63; vs. moral support, 149–65
Moral support, 149–65; natural caring and, 150–53
Moral worth, 60–61
Motility disorders, 38, 40, 43
Mythology, 54–56, 61–63

Nasal cannulas, 121, 122
Nasogastric feeding tube, 70–71, 84, 114, 131, 136
Natural caring, 150–53, 163
Need, response to, in health care policy, 163–64
Neonates, aggressive treatment of, 235, 245
Neutropenia, 71–72
Non-Hodgkin lymphomas, 83
Nurse clinician, 94, 95
Nurses/nursing, 12, 13, 77, 104, 156, 199; delegation of functions of, 216; and home care, 14–15, 16, 25, 181–82; home visits, 75, 87–88; special duty, 200, 206
Nursing agencies, 9–10
Nursing homes, 22, 172, 199, 203, 206, 248; home care vs., 215–16
Nursing services, 207, 208
Nutrition, 67, 70–71, 84, 100–101
Nutritional supplementation, 109, 114–16
Nutritional therapies, 87, 231; cost of, 226, 227

Oncology, 65–78
Opportunistic infections, 79, 80, 82
Opportunity costs, 9, 24, 26, 27, 44, 45, 240, 241, 246, 249

Outpatient care, 72, 73, 76, 82, 88–89, 214
Oxygen supplementation/use, 1, 73, 93, 107, 110, 121–22

Pain control/management, 27, 67, 107, 160; for cancer patients, 69–70; caregivers and, 95–96; for HIV/AIDS patients, 83–84, 87; with PCA, 92, 96, 110, 118
Palliative care, 2, 11, 66, 93, 185, 191, 201, 246–47
Parenteral devices, 93
Parenteral drugs, 96
Parenteral nutrition/feeding, 66, 92, 107, 115–16, 221; Medical coverage for, 207. See also Total parenteral nutrition (TPN)
Parents: elderly, 149, 150–51, 154–55; of technology-dependent children, 42–43, 56–57, 58, 62, 63
Paternalism, 167, 169–72
Patient-controlled analgesia (PCA), 92, 96, 110, 118
Patient management, 10–11
Patient-physician relationship, 13, 75, 184
Patient rights, 108, 171–72, 182, 184
Patients, 12, 27, 213, 224; benefits/burdens of home care, 74–76; control of events, 175; impact of high-tech care on, 4–12; and network of suffering, 161–62; relationship with health care providers, 12–16; right/capacity to make treatment decisions, 185–86; transformations of, 172–74. See also Autonomy (patient); Discharge
Pediatric Home Care Program, 47
Personal care, 7, 136, 157, 202, 204, 216, 221
Personal care agencies, 203–4, 205
Personal care attendant services, 202–3
Personal projects, 155–56, 158
Personality problems, 98–99
Personnel costs, 222
Pharmaceuticals, 207, 208
Physical consequences of home care, 95–99
Physician-assisted suicide, 92–93, 177
Physician services, 208
Physicians: and allocation of expensive technology, 123, 124; and death at home, 176–77; as gatekeepers of technology, 107; hidden costs for, 75; and home care provider responsibilities, 183; home visits, 143, 200; post-death issues, 192, 193; relation-

ship of, with families, 14–15; role of, 12–14, 15–16, 77, 213
Pneumocystis carinii pneumonia (PCP), 72, 80, 82, 87, 221
Post-death issues, 192–93
Pressure sores (decubitus ulcers), 111–13
Preventive treatment, AIDS, 81–82
Pricing issues, 23–24, 214–15, 228–31
Priorities problem, 239, 244, 247
Privacy, 22, 168, 169, 172, 176; family, 12; loss of, 42, 104; and risk of abuse, 171
Private-pay basis, 205
Professional caregiver(s), 157–58. See also Health care professionals
Profit motive, 2, 20, 25, 30, 74, 76, 92
Prognosis, 132, 135, 136, 137–38, 141–42; and caregiver, 153–54
Psychological issues in home care of terminally ill patients, 91–106
Psychological weaning, 101
Psychosocial issues, 17, 85–86, 133, 139–41
Public (the), responsibility of, for health care, 163
Public policy, 23–28, 150, 153, 154
Public policy agenda, 28–29
Public policy recommendations, 193–94
Pumps, portable, 69

Quality, 28, 170; criteria for, 208, 217; issues specific to home care, 212–13, 228; outcomes as indicators for, 211; structure and process measures, 211, 212
Quality assurance, 207, 208–13
Quality-assurance mechanisms, 76, 185–86, 197, 198, 200
Quality of life, 2, 93, 95, 123, 209, 210; for elderly, 109, 122, 123; home care and, 129

Rationing, 27, 121, 160–61, 236, 241–49, 250; criteria, 248–49; with elderly patients, 124; ethically acceptable, 26; prerequisites for fair, 237–41
Regulation/regulatory context, 29, 92, 184–85, 216; absence of, 228, 229–30
Rehospitalization, 138, 139, 144; of elderly patients, 122, 123
Reimbursement(s), 28, 198, 236; through insurance, 76, 230, 231, 248; Medicare beneficiaries, 213–14; physician, 72, 213
Resource allocation, 237, 238, 240–41, 246–48, 250

Resources, limited, competition of technologies for, 238, 240, 241, 244, 246, 249, 250
Respirators, 244; benefits/burdens of, 41–43; efficacy and risks, 35–38
Respiratory care, 67, 73–74, 87; for elderly, 110, 121–24
Respite care, 88, 99, 209, 210
Response-to-need orientation, 149–50, 161, 163–64
Resuscitation, 102, 193
Role reversals, 98
Roles, 6, 8–9, 98, 141, 169–70

Service providers, 204–5; specialized, 205, 206; subsidiary companies, 206. *See also* Health care providers
Services: bundling, 229–30; priorities among, 27–28
Short bowel syndrome, 39–40, 70, 71, 84
Sick room(s), 154, 158–59, 176
Social barriers to use of high-tech health care, 248–49
Social consequences of home care, 95–99
Social costs, 242
Social implications, 1–31, 53, 56–58, 210
Social issues in home care of terminally ill patients, 91–106
Social perspective: and cost containment, 227–28; costs in, 236
Social policy: and pricing issues, 215. *See also* Public policy
Social supports, 86, 87, 193
Social workers, 13, 14–15, 143
Socioeconomic background, 86–87
Specialization, 214; provider, 205, 206
Standards, 28, 29, 197, 198, 208, 228
State laws/policies, 184–85, 192, 228
Stress, 8, 75; caregiver, 44, 95, 123, 139, 200; psychological, 98–99
Structural criteria, 211, 212, 213
Substance abuse, 66, 94, 98
Substituted judgment, principles of, 189, 190
Suffering: and capacity to care, 153–62; network of, 149, 160–62
Support for caregivers/families, 97, 105, 157
Support services/systems, 28, 94
Survivors, 85–86, 176

Team approach, 46, 117, 123, 181–82
Technical supports, 10. *See also* Technology(ies)

Technologically dependent children, 35, 53–64; alternatives to home care, 46–47; effect of, on parents, 42–43, 44; prerequisites to home care, 45–46
Technology(ies), 3, 11, 92, 93; control over, 180; educating caregivers in, 7, 12, 19, 67, 101, 135; in geriatric home care, 109–25; new, 1–2, 107, 224; prerequisites to home care, 67; stress caused by, 8; use of, when no hope of improvement, 43
Terminal care at home, goals of, 93
Terminal illness, 228, 236; benefits/liabilities of high-tech care, 99–105, 100*t*; and exit rights, 172
Terminally ill patients, 91–106, 137–38; rationing care for, 246, 247. *See also* Dying patients
Therapies, 1; with cancer, 65, 66
Third-party payers, 224–25, 231, 236, 242
Total parenteral nutrition (TPN), 4, 6, 27, 35, 67, 221; benefits/burdens of, 41–43, 244; with cancer patients, 71; with children, 45; complications with, 141, 143; costs/charges, 228–29, 229*t*; costs of, 24, 223–24; efficacy and risks, 38–41; with elderly, 109, 114–16, 133–35; errors in, 40; with HIV/AIDS patients, 84, 246–47; reimbursement for, 230
Toxicity, 70, 71, 73, 75
Tracheostomy care, 37, 73, 131, 137
Treatment decisions, 181–82; patient's right/capacity to make, 184, 185–86
Treatment values, 181, 182
Tumors, 65, 66

Urinary tract catherization, 109, 113–14
Utilitarianism, 162, 164

Values, 3, 58–61
Vendors, 9–10, 23–24, 25
Venous access, 93, 117
Ventilator care, 1, 2, 5, 13–14, 45, 122–24, 197, 212, 221, 235; reasons for needing, 36. *See also* Children, ventilator-dependent
Visiting nurses, 87, 201
Visiting Nurse Service, 206, 230

Women, 168; disproportionately burdened, 8–9, 19–21, 136, 161; duty to provide care, 155, 156–57; exploitation of, 149, 156–57